BACKACHE SURVIVAL

OTHER BOOKS BY ROBERT S. IVKER, D.O.

Thriving
Sinus Survival
The Self-Care Guide to Holistic Medicine
Arthritis Survival
Asthma Survival
Headache Survival

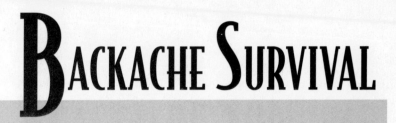

Backache Survival

THE HOLISTIC MEDICAL TREATMENT PROGRAM FOR LOW BACK PAIN

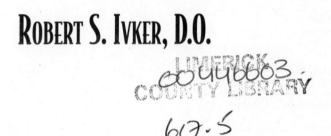

WITHDRAWN FROM STOCK

Robert S. Ivker, D.O.

JEREMY P. TARCHER/PUTNAM
a member of Penguin Group (USA) Inc.
New York

Most Tarcher/Putnam books are available at special quantity discounts for bulk purchase for sales promotions, premiums, fund-raising, and educational needs. Special books or book excerpts also can be created to fit specific needs. For details, write Penguin Group (USA) Inc. Special Markets, 375 Hudson Street, New York, NY 10014.

Jeremy P. Tarcher/Putnam
a member of
Penguin Group (USA) Inc.
375 Hudson Street
New York, NY 10014
www.penguin.com

Library of Congress Cataloging-in-Publication Data

Ivker, Robert S.
    Backache survival : the holistic medical treatment program
for low back pain / Robert S. Ivker.
        p.   cm.
    Includes bibliographical references and index.
    ISBN 1-58542-236-3
        1. Backache—Popular works.   2. Backache—Alternative treatment.
3. Holistic medicine.   I. Title.

RD771.B217I95   2003   2003040183
617.5'6406—dc21

Printed in the United States of America

10   9   8   7   6   5   4   3   2   1

Diagrams by Maude Kernan

To my father-in-law, Irving Goldberg,
for his strength of will in maintaining
a positive attitude and filling the lives
of his loved ones with humor,
in spite of his persistent back pain

ACKNOWLEDGMENTS

I would like to acknowledge Art Brownstein for his many years of pioneering work on himself and his patients in healing back pain naturally. His knowledge and experience, which he generously shared with me, helped pave the way for *Backache Survival*. This book was a team effort comprising the expertise of several gifted healers: Todd Nelson contributed his nutritional knowledge and NLEP; Janna Moll, the energetic and emotional aspects of backache; Anne Day, healing touch; Lawrence Phillips, the Feldenkrais Method; Bob Keck, an inspiring vision of our spiritual evolution; Todd Bezilla, osteopathic medicine; Kathy Fisher, traditional Chinese medicine; and Adam Wagner, chiropractic. A special thanks to two gifted yoga teachers who helped me to identify the most effective yoga postures for treating low back pain—Meredith Vaughn and Shanti Golds-Cousens; and to an exceptional artist—Mandy Kernan Lonergan—who drew the diagrams illustrating these poses.

This is the final book of five in the Survival Guide series, having been preceded by *Sinus, Arthritis, Asthma,* and *Headache Survival,* in addition to *The Self-Care Guide to Holistic Medicine.* I am most grateful to my publisher, Joel Fotinos, for providing me with this opportunity to share the extraordinary health benefits of holistic medicine with many millions of sufferers of our most common chronic conditions. As a holistic family physician for more than thirty years, I continue to be exhilarated by regular emails (through the website: www.sinussurvival.com) from grateful readers. These people have been willing to make the commitment to healing themselves and are thrilled with the results, both with their physical state and in the ways in which the holistic health program has transformed their lives. I would like to acknowledge these individuals who were willing to try this self-care approach and have reaped the rewards. Congratulations! Your feedback, enthusiasm, and energy have fueled every one of the ten books I've written. I would also like to thank my literary agent, Gail Ross, who first suggested the Survival Guide series; Mitch Horowitz, my editor; Allison Sobel; my friends and coauthors of *The Self-Care Guide to Holistic Medicine,* Bob Anderson and Larry Trivieri; and most of all, my wife, Harriet. Her love, support, and patience have helped to make the writing of each of the books an enjoyable experience. I thank God for bringing us together and for compassionately guiding me through the creation of my books and my life!

CONTENTS

BACKACHE SURVIVAL

INTRODUCTION: BACKACHE SURVIVAL

"Only when we are sick of our sickness shall we cease to be sick."

LAO-TZU, FROM THE *TAO TE CHING*

I'd like to begin this book with a "backache" story, one that I know intimately well, because in this case, I became the backache survivor. In August of 2000, my wife and I spent two weeks vacationing in Hawaii. Upon our arrival I was still enjoying the exhilaration from the just completed speaking tour in New Zealand. I had been invited to introduce holistic medicine to this island nation through a series of twelve Sinus Survival seminars and workshops to physicians, health care practitioners, and the public in the five major cities of New Zealand. During the two weeks, I was also interviewed for television, radio, magazines, and newspapers. The fact that this population has the dubious distinction of having the highest incidence of asthma in the world (and no one knows why), and is among the top ten for allergy sufferers, made for a rather intensive, but highly stimulating, trip. I felt very good about what I was able to contribute to help solve their medical mystery and enhance their treatment and prevention of asthma, allergies, and sinusitis. But it was a bit exhausting, and now that I had arrived at this magnificent tropical playground, I was ready for some high-intensity fun.

At the top of my list of favorite activities is hiking. Within the first couple of days, we chose a trail that we had hiked during a previous trip to Hawaii. However, we had been there during the rainy season, and the trail had been very wet and cloaked in low-lying clouds. These conditions had made it somewhat treacherous descending the steep rocky portions of the trail as well as obstructing the spectacular views from the cliffs overlooking the ocean and coastline below that we'd only seen in pictures. But this time we had the perfect cloudless day, and it hadn't rained for several days. The trail and the rocks were dry. I was excited and energized as we set out on the ten-mile loop. It began with a three-mile, 3,000-foot descent to the cliffs, followed by another three miles along the cliff's edge, culminating in a four-mile ascent to the top, not too far from the starting point.

Not infrequently, when I feel this good I'm inspired to indulge myself in one of my greatest thrills—running down very steep trails. This aspect of trail running provides a rush similar to mountain biking down a tortuous trail or skiing an expert slope. You're moving very fast while making a succession of spontaneous and instinctual decisions, often while in midair, on where to place your foot when you land; you're barely on the edge of control, and totally focused. Your mind is completely free of any other thoughts—a type of moving meditation. You're acutely aware that one misstep could result in serious injury, yet the steeper and rockier the trail is, the more fun and the greater the challenge. This trail would prove to be my greatest test—and for my hiking shoes as well. If they didn't hold the rock, then I'd be in big trouble.

After about a half-hour of awesome views and reasonable assurance that the dirt and rocks were dry, I was ready. I told my wife I'd wait for her at the bottom, and I took off (literally). I'd never experienced anything like it before, definitely the most thrilling and frightening trail running I'd ever done. The trail was not only steep and rocky but also narrow and tortuous. As I descended, I very quickly picked up speed. I found myself airborne far more than I was on the ground—leaping from rock to rock or rock to dirt or tree root. While in the air, I'd decide not only where to land but also, if possible, where to go from there. That meant shifting my weight while twisting my body to touch down at the designated spot. It was without a doubt one of the most physically challenging and pleasurable experiences of my life.

But it didn't take long to realize that I'd have to pay a price for this indulgence and that perhaps this was not the best choice of an activity for a 53-year-old guy, even one who is in excellent physical condition. The ten minutes of bliss (which seemed like barely a minute or two) was quickly transformed into three days of back pain. Although I'd treated thousands of patients with the problem, I'd never had the personal experience of incapacitating low back pain. It began gradually while hiking along the relatively flat cliff edge portion of the trail. I attempted to ignore it while appreciating the absolutely incredible scenery surrounding me. The four-mile ascent back up to the top was another story. With almost every increasingly painful step came the messages: "You idiot!" "What a stupid thing to do!" "I've just ruined my one vacation of the year." "I came to a hiker's paradise and this is going to be my first and last hike of the entire two weeks." "I may not even be able to make it up this three-thousand-foot climb." "Harriet might have to hike out alone and get help for me." I was very quickly becoming as miserable as I had been ecstatic just a couple of hours earlier. Fortunately, my worst fears weren't realized, and I was able to make it back to the car. The three days of suffering and miraculous healing that followed provided the bulk of the inspiration for *Backache Survival*.

We returned to the small house we were renting near the beach. I immediately applied a bag of ice cubes to my low back, rubbed in some of the medicinal eucalyptus oil that is a key component of the Sinus Survival Program (it's effective for healing mucous membranes as well as muscle strains), took four ibuprofen tablets, did a couple of gentle stretches, and lay down. When I attempted to get up an hour or so later, I had my first clue of the extent of the damage created by my physical overindulgence. Arising from the bed was a sobering experience and gave me a profound appreciation for the millions of chronic back pain sufferers. It was a painstakingly slow process of progressing from prone to sitting to standing. In those few seconds, with each twinge of acute pain accompanying even the slightest movement, I saw the vision of this long-awaited vacation disappear—hiking, swimming, biking, kayaking, and, most important, making love in one of the most conducive environments on the planet to do so.

The thought occurred to me, "There must be a quick fix to get rid of this pain, relieve the back spasm, and allow me to enjoy myself." But even as I posed the problem, I knew that I was already doing everything I've recommended to patients and nothing had changed. I was also acutely aware that it could possibly be several days before I could get out of bed and simply walk without pain. That outcome, however, came from my conventional medical thinking. In the fifteen years that I'd been practicing holistic medicine, I'd learned that anything is possible. Miracles, and spontaneous healing, can occur on a regular basis. Not only do you have to open your mind to that possibility, but you can help to facilitate that outcome if you focus on identifying the emotional factors that almost always contribute to triggering the physical problem. If these issues are addressed, expressed, and accepted, then you'll increase your chances considerably of more quickly healing your body. It's what I'd taught my patients for years: "Allow yourself to feel your feelings"; "Your issues are held in your tissues." But now that I was the patient, I was reminded of how challenging a process that emotional work is. You become so consumed with the pain and physical disability and the more superficial feelings associated with them—anger (*"I did this to myself by making such a bad decision"*), sadness (*"My vacation is ruined"*), and guilt (*"I've spoiled it for my wife, too"*)— that it becomes quite a challenge to go beyond these feelings to the underlying emotions that preceded the onset of the pain.

Since the mid-'80s when I began practicing holistic medicine, I'd observed the connection between sinusitis and repressed anger both within myself and in so many of my patients. However, in recent years I've become increasingly fascinated with a deeper level of the mind-body connection. It's been nothing short of astounding to see the correlation between a wide variety of very specific physical symptoms and their corresponding mental/emotional issues. What several of the leading contemporary pioneers in this aspect of holistic medicine have uncovered is something that has been well known for thousands of years in both traditional Chinese and Ayurvedic (traditional Indian) medicine. Each of the seven primary chakras (literally "spinning wheel"; they form the basis of Ayurvedic medicine) is associated with several mental and emotional issues. (This is also true of each of the body's organs in traditional Chinese medicine.) When there is physical pain or an ailment, it usually indicates a weakness or an obstruction of the flow of energy through the particular chakra closest to the dysfunctional body part. I realize now that physical pain is for the most part a reflection of emotional pain. The painful feelings, however, are often so deep that we are not even aware of them. Men, especially, usually require significant physical discomfort to help them become more conscious of their underlying painful emotions. Unfortunately, though, in most instances, they still don't get the message or take the opportunity to heal at a deeper level or to prevent recurrence of the physical problem. Most people, just as I was doing with my incapacitating backache, opt for the quick fix (assuming there is one) and spend all of their time and energy focused on the obvious but superficial aspect of their problem. They usually learn very little from their painful ordeal. I was determined not to allow that to happen to me, although I could very easily see how I could follow that same route. But since I had already spent one day trying all of the "quick fixes" I knew, and none of them seemed to be working, I decided to opt for the holistic route.

In the case of low back pain, there is often an overlap of the first (root) and second (sacral) chakras. Backs represent support, and the mental/emotional issues often associated with low back pain have to do with a lack of financial support; security; groundedness—a feeling of connection with nature and the Earth; a sense of connection to your tribe or family; blame and guilt; sex; and one-on-one relationships, usually with a woman. Knowing that one or more of these issues had significantly contributed to my backache, and since I wasn't aware of any emotional pain, I began to reflect on my life as I lay immobile in our cottage throughout the day following the traumatic hike. I got up only to go to the bathroom. And as painful as that was, I wasn't surprised at how infrequent those short trips were.

During the six months prior to my arrival in Hawaii, I had experienced both exhilaration and significant insecurity. I had completed the manuscripts for the fourth edition of *Sinus Survival* and its first offspring, *Arthritis Survival*. And although I felt great pride in the finished product, I wasn't sure how *Arthritis* would be received by my editor (I'd just sent it in before leaving for New Zealand) or by the public. Even more important, I was way behind on my writing schedule and knew that I would never make the contractual deadline the publisher had set for *Asthma Survival*. When I agreed to take on this five-book Survival Guide series, I'd decided to temporarily suspend my medical practice to allow enough time for writing. That left my wife and me largely dependent on the book income (advances) to support ourselves. It was a bit of a risk, but as long as I met the deadlines and received the installments as scheduled, we should be O.K. But if I was not able to complete the manuscripts on time, I might have to forfeit that income and lose the opportunity to write the remaining books. Although I didn't dwell on it constantly, I knew it was always there lurking in the not-so-deep recesses of my mind.

The other major development in my life that year occurred six months earlier, when Bob Anderson (president of the American Board of Holistic Medicine [ABHM]) and I agreed to move forward with the creation of the first board certification examination, along with the first board review course in holistic medicine. Since co-founding (along with twelve other holistic physicians) the ABHM in 1996, our initial objective was to create a certification exam to establish a standard of care for holistic medicine. We determined that we needed at least $60,000 to launch this project and do it properly. Early in 2000, even though we had only raised $20,000, we decided that the time was right and that we should go ahead and just borrow the money we needed for the initial expenses. We hoped that registration fees for both the course and exam would then cover the remainder of the considerable expense required for both events. When I arrived in Hawaii, the brochures announcing the course and exam had just been mailed out. Although we'd had some early indication of a positive response, I was still feeling considerable insecurity even though I hadn't really acknowledged it. (This historic event subsequently attracted 425 participants—physicians and health care practitioners from all fifty states, and nearly 300 M.D.s and D.O.s sat for the first certification exam. It was a success in every sense of the word.) And although I consider myself an optimist, in early August, four months before the main event, I was feeling considerable insecurity.

Another possible contributor to my back pain was the fact that periods of insecurity are often accompanied by a lack of closeness in my marriage. I had been overly consumed with my work for a prolonged period, and intimacy had suffered as a result.

Although my time in bed was not exactly what I'd had in mind when I began the vacation, the opportunity it provided me for this introspection had proven to be quite useful. I'd identified several instances of financial insecurity, a perceived lack of support, and a disconnection from my wife with associated guilt and blame, each one an emotional factor that might have contributed to my physical pain. I expressed these feelings to my wife, in addition to writing and journaling about them during day two of my recovery. By the end of that second day, I had also created affirmations that addressed my painful emotions, for example, "I am safe and secure"; "I trust the process of life." These were accompanied by healing visualizations, and by the next morning there was enough improvement (arising from bed was my most effective gauge) that I was able to go for a short walk, albeit with moderate pain. The holistic approach and the diminished pain I experienced as a result of releasing some of this emotional pain convinced me that the cumulative effect of all of these issues was the primary cause of my being physically incapacitated. And that it was a far more significant factor than having used my spine as a shock absorber as I flew down the trail, even though that was clearly the trigger. I was pleased with my progress and encouraged that we might still be able to stick with our original plan, which was to hike the next morning on our favorite trail to a place we'd never been before but which had been highly recommended. It's a rugged path that winds along the cliffs above the ocean for two miles and then climbs inland for another two miles to a spectacular waterfall. But realistically I still had a long way to go before I'd be ready for something that strenuous. So I decided to call a friend who lives on the island, who just happens to be a certified Healing Touch practitioner. By late in the afternoon of the third day, as I got up from Leilani's treatment table, I could immediately tell that there was significant improvement. That's when I knew that I was ready to attempt the hike the following day.

We awoke the next morning before dawn, planning to be at the trailhead by daybreak. It still was far from a pain-free experience getting out of bed that morning. But I was determined to go and enjoy this hike. And I did. But I sure had my doubts early on, as we made our way up and down over rocks, tree roots, and small streams, continually climbing and dropping several hundred feet while traversing some of the most beautiful terrain on the planet. Unfortunately, however, this was obviously not the best method for rehabilitating my back. The pain was moderate in intensity and grabbed my attention as well as the muscles in my low back throughout most of the four miles in. Along the way, I was conscious of breathing abdominally to relax the muscles and repeating the affirmations to myself that I'd created two days earlier. Both of these techniques were helpful in distracting my mind and shifting the focus away from the pain, even allowing me to enjoy the experience for at least some of the time.

As we approached our final destination, I was beginning to feel some concern about the four-mile return trip and what impact that would have on my back. And then as we climbed around a big bend in the trail we got our first glimpse of the most magnificent waterfall I'd ever seen. A few minutes later we were close enough to begin to hear the falls striking the pool below. And then we arrived. It's difficult to describe the magical feel of this incredible spot as I looked up at the falls. Although they were much too high to see the top from this vantage point, I could strongly feel their power, their awe-inspiring beauty, the surrounding lush vegetation, the sheer dark-gray volcanic rock walls, and the large crystal clear pool at the base. My wife and I had left early enough to have the opportunity to experience this special place by ourselves. The sun was not yet high enough to reach this hidden oasis, so it was quite cool. And although the water was even cooler, I felt drawn, almost magnetized, to come even closer. I took off my clothes and entered what felt to me like a sacred pool; it was almost like approaching an altar (and a very cold one at that). Although I was somewhat mesmerized, my back instantly reminded me that cold water is not usually the best remedy for eliminating back pain. (Hot tubs and moist heat are typically recommended.) I swam slowly toward the falls, then under them to a cave just behind. As I sat there naked on my knees just at the edge of the cave with the water falling on my head and shoulders, it was as if I was completely immersed in the womb of Mother Earth. I began to meditate and recite the affirmations. Then I prayed and asked God, Gaia (the earth goddess), all the nature spirits, and my spirit guides to help me to heal my back. Within two to three minutes I felt the pain dissipate, and after about five minutes under the falls I slowly swam back to shore totally pain-free. I had just personally experienced a miracle—a spontaneous healing. I've helped many patients to experience spiritual healing through the modality of healing touch, but I'd never been the recipient. I had just been touched by the hand of God, and it was one of the most powerful and exhilarating experiences of my life. I got out of the water and excitedly reported to my wife that my back was completely better.

The hike back was more enjoyable than I can even describe. The back pain was gone, and it has never returned. My personal experience with this episode of acute low back pain and the way in which it was healed are the inspiration for this book and serve as the basis for the Backache Survival Program. I don't intend for you to have to go to Hawaii and sit under a waterfall, but most of the components of this holistic approach can be applied anywhere. As long as you're willing to make the commitment to healing your life, you have an excellent chance of living without chronic back pain. Good luck, be patient and persistent, and enjoy yourself.

Rob Ivker
January 2003

Chapter 1

THE BACKACHE "QUICK FIX"

Backache, regardless of whether it's acute or chronic, is a message your body is sending you that there is an imbalance in your life. The practice of holistic medicine restores your balance while addressing each aspect of your life—body, mind, and spirit—and utilizes both conventional and complementary therapies to prevent and treat disease. Most important, the focus of holistic medicine is on creating a state of optimal well-being. The goal of *Backache Survival* is for you to learn to use the symptom of back pain to transform your experience toward physical, environmental, mental, emotional, spiritual, and social fitness. To create this condition of holistic health, the *causes* of back pain are treated just as aggressively as the physical *symptoms*. If you become an attentive observer of the triggers of your backache (and this book will assist you in this training), you will learn a great deal, not only about the causes of your back pain but also about the nature of the imbalance in your life. You will become much more effective at treating, as well as preventing, your backache. The primary therapeutic modality in mitigating the multiple factors responsible for causing backache is *love*. The fundamental principle underlying America's newest specialty is: *Unconditional love is life's most powerful healer;* and its corollary is: The primary cause of chronic disease is the *deprivation of love.* This book will help guide you in a process of learning to love and nurture your back, along with the rest of your body, your mind, and your spirit, while simultaneously offering you many options for quickly relieving and preventing backache.

I have spent the majority of my time during the past fifteen years treating a variety of chronic conditions and helping my patients experience optimal health as they heal their lives. Most have come to see me after reading one of my books and typically after also seeing one or more physicians who were unsuccessful in providing them with a long-term conventional medical quick fix for their ailment. Medication, and often surgery as well, gave them only temporary relief. Although most of these people didn't admit it, they arrived at my office hoping for an alternative quick fix to relieve their chronic pain. That might well have been your motivation to buy this book. Even though miracles and spontaneous healings are certainly possible, for the vast majority of sufferers of *chronic* back pain there is *no quick fix*. Remember, the story that I just related in the Introduction, of my own healing was an *acute* episode of back pain. I had not been in pain for months or years, as many of you have. But I do strongly believe that if you closely adhere to the recommendations in chapters 4, 5, and 6 (many of which are introduced in this chapter), you will see a significant if not dramatic improvement in your condition within two to three months. (The therapies mentioned in this chapter are those that produce the quickest results.) There is a big difference between acute relief and long-term correction of the underlying causes. I want you to both feel better as soon as possible and prevent further suffering later on. This approach is remarkably effective at both treating and preventing almost any chronic condition.

Bear in mind as you begin to implement this holistic treatment program that true healing is far greater than simply the absence of pain or illness. The most effective way to cure any chronic condition is to *heal your life,* not just repair your physical dysfunction, which in your case is backache.

I realize that, when embarking on a life-changing program requiring a strong personal commitment, most people in our society would like a simple and safe way to take the initial step. To facilitate change, you must first lessen the resistance that may arise from your anticipation of how much time you will need to invest in this program. If it is a high enough priority, you will be willing to take the time. You may also need to modify your attitude toward approaching regular exercise, long-term dietary changes, as well as taking dietary supplement pills on a regular basis. In addition, you might be confronting the fear of letting go of long-held beliefs and behaviors that have dictated the way you live your life. This insecurity is perfectly understandable and appropriate. Therefore, rather than trying to do everything at once, which for many people can be overwhelming, this chapter will offer you several options for experiencing relatively rapid *symptom improvement* while *gradually* introducing this holistic approach into your life. Although the focus of the book is on chronic low back pain, many of the recommendations in this and the following chapters can be of help with both acute and chronic back pain.

The primary objective of the Backache Survival Program and the holistic treatment for any chronic disease is to heal the specific part of the body that is not functioning properly. The method for correcting this physical dysfunction is for you to nurture not only the diseased part but your entire body, including your mind and spirit.

This healing process usually begins on the physical level because the body provides the most immediate feedback: telling you what makes you feel better and what makes you feel worse. But if you're feeling some degree of backache all the time, it's not easy to determine what one intervention—a stretching exercise, herb, postural change, or relaxation technique—is doing for you. It has usually taken many months or years to produce the conditions creating your ongoing problem with backache. Therefore, it will take some time for your body to function well enough on a consistent basis for you to begin to trust the signals and feedback it is giving you. By improving physically at the outset, you'll become much more aware of what you can do to heighten this feeling of well-being and what behaviors—how much you're sleeping, how you're exercising, what you're eating, what's eating you—make you feel worse. Over time you will learn to become your own best healer and develop reference points for what techniques work best for you.

To speed the process of correcting the imbalances in your life, I have developed the initial Physical and Environmental Health Components of the Backache Survival Program, many of which are included in the list of "quick-fix" suggestions. It won't be effortless, but if you're committed to healing and curing your backache, this is the most effective way to begin. This approach will enable you to feel better as quickly as possible. You can begin your training as a healer of backache by initially following the recommendations in this chapter; gaining a greater understanding of what causes backache in Chapter 2; and taking the Wellness Self-Test in Chapter 3. That will prepare you to make a stronger commitment to the Backache Survival Program in Chapter 4. Chapters 4, 5, and 6 will help you to understand *why* all of the recommendations are included (I have page references for most of them) and better appreciate how they are helping your back and enhancing your health.

I've found that if you stay on the complete regimen described in this chapter for at least four to eight weeks, you will usually be able to at least partially restore physical balance and experience considerable and often dramatic improvement. You should also be able to decrease the use of analgesics and any other medication you're presently taking for back pain. The physical and environmental health recommendations are explained in more depth in Chapter 4, mental and emotional in Chapter 5, and spiritual and social in Chapter 6. The improvement in your physical condition will usually provide the motivation to commit to and fully benefit from the mind and spirit components of the program while addressing all of the causes of your ailment.

The Backache Survival Program will enlighten and educate you: You'll learn why you've suffered for so long and what you can do to improve that condition. But for this treatment program to make a profound difference in your life, you'll need to give yourself a gentle but firm push in the direction of optimal health—a condition of high energy and vitality, creativity, peace of mind, self-awareness, self-acceptance, passion, and intimacy. The critical ingredients for your success are a heightened *awareness* of your needs and desires (What do you want your life to be like?); a *commitment* to providing them for yourself; the *time* required to incorporate new healthy habits into your life; and the *discipline* to stay on your course in spite of episodes of significant pain. These are the essential factors in learning to love and nurture yourself, and especially your aching back. And it is also the primary objective of this holistic medical treatment program.

If you are willing to make the commitment, this program will enable you to *heal yourself of backache.* Although you might still have occasional episodes of back pain, they will occur less frequently, won't be as incapacitating or last as long as they do now, nor will they require your ongoing dependence on medication. More important, you will understand why the backache occurred, have the tools to treat it quickly, and avoid the debilitating and frightening experience of enduring such severe pain that you are unable to function for a prolonged period of time. Keep in mind that the most significant aspect of your healing process is that, through your pain, you will almost always learn or relearn a valuable lesson that helps to *prevent* subsequent backaches.

Although optimal health requires a commitment to a lifelong healing *process,* we obviously live in an age of the quick fix. We've grown up believing that there's a fast and effortless solution to all of life's hardships. And if there is no such miracle available today, it won't be long before science and technology provide it. But healing your dysfunctional back, while creating a balance of optimal well-being throughout every dimension of your life, requires a commitment to the Backache Survival Program comparable to one you would make if you'd just started a new job. *Healing yourself is the most important work you'll ever do, and the greatest gift you'll ever receive.*

After two months of making a commitment to this program, you will probably be "surviving" quite well, with a significant improvement in your symptoms. If you can maintain and strengthen that commitment to yourself, within six months you will be healthier than you've been in years, and within one year you'll be experiencing a state of well-being you've never known before. The most important advice I can give you is to take your time, be gentle and accepting of yourself, and know that there are no mistakes—only lessons. Study diligently, listen attentively, be willing to take risks, and have fun while you're at it. It's definitely a challenge, but the rewards are unimaginable.

In the list that follows, *one asterisk* in the left margin—next to the recommendations, vitamins, and supplements that can be started at the outset—denotes *stage one* (physical and environmental). *Two asterisks* denote the *second stage* (mental and emotional), which you can begin three weeks later. The *third stage,* marked by *three asterisks,* begins after another three weeks (social and spiritual). You have the option of doing and taking everything right from the beginning or at any time of your choosing, and simply following the instructions in the table. If it's too much for you, your body—and especially your back—will tell you. The only significant risk that I'm aware of in starting out with the entire list is that it may feel a bit overwhelming and too much of a challenge to *maintain* the new daily practices rather than if you gradually ease into it. If you would like to proceed even more slowly, which is perfectly fine to do, then I suggest the following: After about two months of incorporating most of the physical and environmental health recommendations into your daily routine (the single-asterisk items), you can begin the mental and emotional health components of the program (two asterisks), followed in another one to two months by social and spiritual health (three asterisks). Each of the different therapeutic options presented will contribute some benefit. There is no single remedy or magic potion that will quickly cure your chronic back pain, but the following therapies work more quickly than anything else I'm aware of in treating backache. Many of the products included in the quick-fix list that are not readily available at most health food stores can be obtained by referring to the Product Index at the end of the book. There are many options available to you other than those on this list. Please read chapters 4, 5, and 6 thoroughly, and you may find some others that you prefer.

With each component of the Essential 8 program, you will

be uncovering factors that have contributed to causing your backache. Remember, the more often you experience a sense of physical well-being, the more acutely aware you'll become of what makes you feel good and what triggers the episodes of pain. This information initially will allow you to make healthier choices regarding how much and how well you're stretching, exercising, breathing, sitting, eating, and drinking. As you progress, you'll find that the latter four aspects of health—comprising the *mind* and *spirit* sections—require far less of your time but a deeper commitment and greater awareness than the recommendations for the *body*. However, the more you can work on these less tangible but potentially more health-enhancing factors, you will be able to effectively *prevent* severe attacks of backache, *reduce* or *eliminate* your analgesics and medications, and possibly *cure* yourself of chronic low back pain.

THE QUICK-FIX BACKACHE SURVIVAL PROGRAM

★(1) Ice—apply only after an injury or acute back pain, and for no more than 48 hours. Fill a plastic bag with ice cubes, then wrap the bag in a moist towel. Place the wrapped bag on your back and leave in place for 20 minutes, then re-apply hourly for 20 minutes.

★(2) Lie on floor on your back with feet and calves elevated on a chair with knees at right angle to the floor. For relief of acute muscle spasm.

★(3) Heating pad, hot shower, shower massager with moderate pressure, Jacuzzi, or hot tub for acute pain that persists beyond 48 hours; and for chronic pain. Follow this with yoga or stretching.

★(4) Apply arnica cream and/or take arnica tablets.

★(5) Analgesics—Tylenol, ibuprofen (Advil, Nuprin), naproxen (Aleve), or aspirin. All are equally effective for pain relief, but Tylenol does not have an anti-inflammatory effect.

★(6) Herbal Muscle Relief—2 tablets 3 to 5 times a day (page 124).

★(7) Gluteal squeezes—lie on your back with your knees

bent and your feet flat on the bed or floor; squeeze the muscles in your buttocks as tightly as you can, then slowly relax. Works well for both acute and chronic pain.

(8) Yoga or stretching—this is probably the single best therapy for chronic low back pain. Begin gradually with gentle stretches (page 133).

★(9) Drink more water—bottled or filtered; ½ oz. per lb. of body weight (page 78).

★(10) Practice abdominal breathing for at least 5 minutes, 2 times a day (page 74).

★(11) Begin walking (if you're not already doing so) for at least 20 minutes, 4 to 5 times a week (page 147).

★(12) Make sure your workplace is ergonomically sound, and practice good posture. Avoid sitting for prolonged periods of time; if it can't be avoided, then stand and/or take a brief walk every 15 to 20 minutes (page 144).

★(13) Sleep on a firm mattress for at least 7 to 9 hours per night (page 161).

★(14) Collagen Support—2 tablets morning and night.

★(15) Super Potency Essential Fatty Acids—2 capsules 2 to 3 times a day with meals to reduce inflammation (pages 104 and 122).

★(16) Herbal Joint Relief—for acute pain: 2 tablets 4 times a day on an empty stomach; chronic and maintenance dosage: 2 tablets morning and night on an empty stomach to reduce inflammation (page 125).

★(17) Glucosamine CarePlus—2 tablets 3 times a day to reduce pain, promote joint health, and reduce arthritis in the spine (page 119).

★(18) Calcium Supreme—2 tablets 3 times a day with meals (page 119).

★(19) Magnesium Extra—2 tablets at breakfast and dinner (page 119).

★(20) Apply a medicinal eucalyptus oil and/or capsaicin (cayenne) cream (menthol-based) to your back.

★(21) Professional care therapies:
  ★(a) Physician (M.D. or D.O.)—for injection of long-acting anesthetic into site of pain. Precision of diagnosis is key to successful treatment. In the hands of a highly skilled practitioner, this can be an extremely effective treatment for acute pain (page 165).
  ★(b) Healing Touch—highly therapeutic for both acute and chronic pain (page 163).
  ★(c) Craniosacral therapy—a type of osteopathic manipulative therapy (OMT) that works very well for both acute and chronic pain (page 168).
  ★(d) Chiropractic—can be helpful in treating both acute and chronic low back pain (page 171).
  ★(e) Massage therapy—excellent for temporary relief (page 176).
  ★(f) Acupuncture—works for both acute and chronic pain, short- and long-term relief (page 173).
  ★(g) Trigger point therapy—either deep pressure or injections of anesthetic to chronically sore areas (page 164).
  ★★(h) Biofeedback—works well for chronic pain and is not difficult to learn (page 215).
★★(22) Practice affirmations and visualizations (pages 196 and 210).
★★(23) Do emotional release work on a regular basis—express feelings to a spouse, partner, close friend, or psychotherapist (page 209); journaling (page 228); anger release (page 225).
★★(24) Laugh more and learn to take things less seriously (page 215).
★★★(25) Pray and practice gratitude daily (page 243).
★★★(26) Spend time daily on building intimacy—communication, physical intimacy, recreation (page 257).
★★★(27) Practice forgiveness and start with yourself (page 271).

Chapter 2

WHAT IS BACKACHE? WHAT CAUSES IT? HOW DOES CONVENTIONAL MEDICINE TREAT IT?

PREVALENCE

According to the National Center for Health Statistics, backache is the seventh most common chronic condition in the United States, afflicting approximately 20 million people. This is the number of *chronic* sufferers, but backache is a problem that nearly 80 percent of Americans (220 million) will experience at some point in their lives, mostly on an acute basis. The vast majority of these backache sufferers have *low back pain,* which is the focus of *Backache Survival.* (It is estimated that 80 percent of back pain treated in doctors' offices is in the lower lumbar [low back] region, with 20 percent in the neck and thoracic [midback] area. When I use the term "backache" throughout the book, I am referring to low back pain, unless I state otherwise.) Fortunately, most of the 220 million, like myself, will have only an acute episode of pain and suffer for a relatively short period of time. Unfortunately, more than half the people who recover from a first episode of acute low back pain will have a recurrence within a few years. And although most instances of back pain resolve on their own within two to four weeks, about 10 percent will persist beyond four to six weeks. I'm assuming that the vast majority of you are reading this book because you're among this latter group of chronic sufferers (with occasional acute flare-ups)—those who have been dealing with the problem for many months or years.

If it's of any comfort to you, you're not alone. Backache is the number-one cause of disability in the United States for people under the age of 45, and the second (to the common cold) most common cause of absence from the workplace among people younger than 55. It is estimated that 50 million working days are lost each year due to back pain, and $50 billion is spent annually to treat the problem. This figure includes the nearly 250,000 back surgeries performed annually but does not include disability or workmen's compensation payments. Backache is the second most frequently cited reason for visiting a medical clinic (accounting for 13 million visits to primary care physicians' offices each year) and the sixth most common reason for visiting an emergency room. While 79 percent of patients with acute low back pain will see one physician (typically their family doctor), 21 percent will see multiple practitioners, including chiropractors, orthopedic surgeons, neurosurgeons, psychiatrists, rheumatologists, and physical therapists. The cost of seeing multiple health care specialists is generally four times the cost of seeing one primary care physician. More than half of low back patients who have suffered for at least three months will seek out multiple practitioners for help. Backache can strike people of all ages, but usually not before the teenage years, and becomes more common between the ages of 30 and 50 as the intervertebral discs lose some of their ability to absorb shock and as backs become more unstable from inactivity. It is slightly more common in males. Interestingly, backache is far more common in sedentary societies. Native peoples like the Australian aborigines, the Masai tribe and the Bushman of Africa, or in the countries of India, China, Japan, or the Philippines where people spend little time sitting in prolonged positions of flexion (forward bending) have very little back pain.

ANATOMY AND PHYSIOLOGY

The back encompasses the entire length of the body from the neck to the tailbone and is divided into cervical (neck), thoracic, lumbar, sacral, and coccygeal areas (the low back refers to the

21

latter three). The back is closely connected in some way to nearly every other part of the body, but most directly with the shoulders, arms, legs, pelvis, and hips. Although we often think of the back as a single entity, it is actually a complex connection of *many parts.* These include:

• *Bones,* including the spinal column, consisting of twenty-four movable bones (the vertebrae), and nine relatively fixed bones making up the sacrum and coccyx, or tailbone. The sacrum and coccyx rest between the bones of the pelvis and the back. The pelvic bones themselves are also considered part of the back.

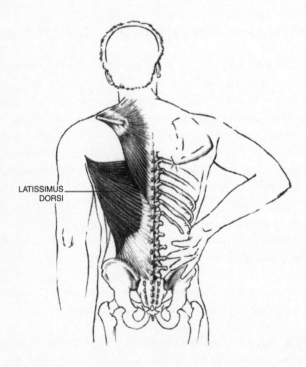

LATISSIMUS
DORSI

Figure 2.1   *Back Anatomy*

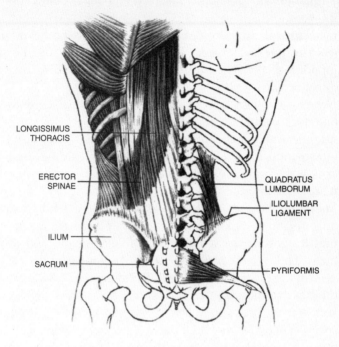

FIGURE 2.2 *Lower Back Anatomy*

- *Intervertebral discs* are cartilaginous, fluid-filled shock absorbers, located between all of the vertebrae.
- *Nerves* of the low back, which include a pair of nerves that leave the spinal cord at each level, one on each side below each vertebra. These later join together to form the nerves of the low back, the pelvis, and the legs. Several nerves come together in the buttocks and run down the back of each leg as the sciatic nerve. This nerve later divides and innervates the entire leg all the way to the tips of the toes.
- *Muscles,* which connect the spine and pelvis to the lower back and the upper back as well as the ribs, hips, abdomen, and legs.
- *Ligaments,* which form static supports between the vertebrae, sacrum, and pelvic bones.

The functions of these different structures are as follows:

- *Bones* provide support and form for the entire body and protect the internal organs. The spinal column is flexible and supports the weight of the head while also protecting the spinal cord.
- *Nerves* carry signals from the brain and spinal cord to the muscles to allow for movement, sensation of pain and pleasure, heat and cold, pressure, and sharpness. They also send information back to the nervous system regarding the position of the body, how far it is bent, how fast it is moving, and where it is in space.
- *Muscles* perform various movements, including bending, squatting, rotating, walking, standing, sitting, and rising up. The muscles govern the spine's curvature, alignment, and movement. They are the most important component of the back in determining its relative strength, flexibility, and health. Due to the fact that most pain receptors are found in the muscles (the vertebrae and discs have almost no pain receptors), *back pain originates in the muscles.* Back muscles are highly sensitive to pain due to the proximity of the spinal cord. There are four layers of muscles in the spine that participate in the highly complex movements of the spine and also help to maintain posture. As a result of its muscular interconnections, the spine can be affected by dysfunction in other parts of the body.
- *Ligaments* hold the vertebrae together in their linear alignment. Together with the *intervertebral discs,* they assist the spinal column with flexion (forward bending), extension (back bending), and lateral flexion (side bending); and support it from lateral and compression forces.

Together, all of these parts of the back allow us to do a variety of activities, to comfortably remain in one position, to balance ourselves, and to perform very complex movements. The nervous system also helps coordinate various motions so that the different muscles and joints in a particular area work together to allow for coordinated movements and actions.

SYMPTOMS AND DIAGNOSIS

"Backache" is the term used to describe a variety of conditions. Your symptoms, a thorough medical history, and a physical exam are the major components in establishing a diagnosis. However, the major problem in effectively treating backache is the difficulty in making a diagnosis. According to R. Deyo, M.D., the leading medical researcher on this subject, "Up to 85 percent of patients with low back pain cannot be given a definitive diagnosis because of the poor association among symptoms, pathologic findings, and imaging results." This situation exists primarily because there are very few conventional physicians who are well trained in evaluating the low back and able to make a clear diagnosis. The bulk of their training and physical examination is spent ruling out herniated discs, which are present in fewer than 5 percent of the patients with low back pain. The physical examination in most cases of backache reveals excessive muscle tightness and spasm, along with significant limitation of motion in all directions—flexion, extension, and lateral flexion. X rays typically show no abnormalities with both acute and chronic backache (helpful only for ruling out the more serious causes of back pain, e.g., tumors or TB), and, as Deyo mentions, even the more high-tech diagnostic tools, such as MRI (magnetic resonance imaging), are often not very helpful in making a definitive diagnosis. In fact, the MRI is known to be inaccurate 10 to 20 percent of the time. Yet thousands of painful and expensive surgical procedures are performed every year based on the results of MRIs that show spinal disc abnormalities ("slipped discs"). This practice has continued despite a 1994 study that focused on the use of MRIs and appeared in the *New England Journal of Medicine.* It found no correlation between structural abnormalities (revealed on MRIs) and back pain. This study was based in part on the finding that among ninety-eight people *without* back pain, two thirds had spinal abnormalities, including herniated, bulging, or protruding intervertebral discs; discs with minor "degenerative joint changes"; and flattened, narrowed discs, especially at the L5-S1 level. All are common on

MRI scans, especially in older people. One third of these people had more than one disc abnormality, yet none had experienced any back pain. These findings may create unnecessary anxiety for the patient and could lead to further testing and procedures, including surgery. But if spinal stenosis or a severe nerve injury is suspected following the physical exam (symptoms may include the loss of reflexes and true muscle weakness), then an MRI may be warranted.

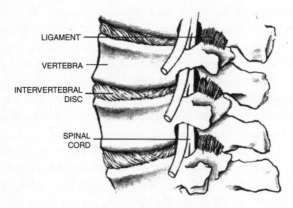

FIGURE 2.3   *Normal Lumbar Spine*

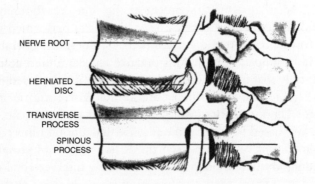

FIGURE 2.4   *Lumbar Spine with Herniated Disc*

In spite of Deyo's dismal statistics, there is an excellent chance for a well-trained physician to make a *definitive diagnosis.* Most osteopathic physicians are highly skilled in doing a structural exam and evaluating the back, especially those who have maintained their skills in osteopathic manipulative treatment (OMT). A thorough history will include a careful accounting of all your symptoms: the type of pain, its location and duration, body positions that relieve or aggravate the pain, activities you were engaged in just before the onset of the pain, and the current stressors affecting your life. People with chronic low back pain will invariably attribute the onset of the pain to a physical event— an injury, automobile accident, or lifting a heavy object. However, a good holistic health history (refer to Chapter 3 and the Wellness Self-Test) will usually reveal significant stressful factors, often including financial stress, a divorce, or some other emotionally traumatic event that might have preceded the onset of backache. This evaluation, coupled with a careful, well-focused physical examination, is often all that's necessary to make a diagnosis. In one study on two hundred patients with workmen's compensation injuries of the low back, performed by Neil Nathan, M.D., a holistic family physician, it was found that more than 80 percent had localized their pain to one or both of the sacroiliac joints. Less common injuries included that of the spinal ligaments, muscles (especially the pyriformis, gluteus, quadratus lumborum, and psoas), iliolumbar ligaments, facet joints, ribs, and, last, the protruding disc (accounting for only 3.2 percent of the patients). If Dr. Nathan suspects an injured sacroiliac joint injury, he'll often inject the joint with an anesthetic and perform OMT (see page 165). About 70 percent of these patients are completely better within one week, while 30 percent will require a second injection. He repeatedly makes the point "that precision of diagnosis is the key to effective treatment."

With the less common causes listed in item 6 below, there will usually be symptoms that are more systemic (the whole body is affected) and less localized to the back. A good example would be weight loss, which is often seen in both tuberculosis and cancer.

Although the exact diagnosis is not often determined, the possibile diagnoses include the following:

(1) *Sprain* and *strain,* often used interchangeably, are the most prevalent forms of low back pain. A strain is usually an overstretched muscle, and a sprain a partially torn ligament, but in most cases of backache it isn't clear which one it is.

(2) *Muscle spasm* is a painful, sustained, and involuntary contraction of muscles in the back.

(3) *Osteoarthritis,* or arthritis of the joints of the spine (also called "spondylitis"), is a common consequence of aging and is present in nearly all individuals over the age of 75, though not all experience back pain as a result. *Ankylosing spondylitis* is a far more serious and painful arthritic condition of the spine.

(4) *Herniated disc,* or "slipped disc," accounts for only 2 to 4 percent of backaches. In actuality, the disc *herniates,* or bulges, between two vertebrae and may eventually rupture. This bulging disc may push against a spinal nerve, causing shooting pains, tingling, or numbness to extend into the leg. Most often, the affected spinal nerve is the sciatic, the largest one, and when that occurs the condition is called *sciatica.* (Sciatica is discussed separately in item 7 below.)

(5) *Structural problems* include kyphosis, scoliosis, and spinal stenosis (see item 8 below).

(6) *Underlying medical conditions,* such as kidney pain (including kidney stones), spinal tumor, spinal tuberculosis (Pott's disease), or metastatic prostate cancer, account for a small percentage of backache.

(7) *Sciatica* refers to aching or pain along the route of the sciatic nerve, the largest and longest nerve in the body. It is actually a group of nerves encased in a sheath. The right and left branches of the sciatic nerve extend from the base of the spinal cord through the buttocks and the back of each thigh to the knee, where it branches and extends down into the feet. Sciatica most often affects people in

their forties and fifties. The irritation of the sciatic nerve usually results from compression of the nerve from bulging, herniating, ruptured, or torn discs, in addition to scar tissue from prior surgeries and spinal stenosis. Sciatica often presents with the following symptoms:

- Pain in the low back, lower buttock, or back of the leg, which may radiate down to the foot; can be either mild and intermittent, or severe and persistent. Pain is usually worse with movement, laughing, sneezing, coughing, straining with a bowel movement, and at night.
- Muscle spasms, weakness, numbness, or tingling (pins and needles) in buttock or leg.
- As a result of the chronic pain, other symptoms may include severe fatigue, inability to sleep, irritability and increased anger, and loss of ability to perform typical activities of daily living. Sometimes, severe depression can also be present, including feelings of extreme sadness and hopelessness, crying spells, insomnia, and loss of appetite. These symptoms can occur even without a prior history of depression and should be treated by a physician. In about half of all cases of sciatica, the pain resolves spontaneously within four weeks.

(8) *Spinal stenosis* is a narrowing in the spinal canal due to soft tissue, scar tissue, or bony tissue impingement. If severe, this can result in nerve compression. *Foraminal stenosis* is impingement on the nerve roots where they exit the spinal cord through the neural foramina in the vertebrae. This can be due to soft tissue encroachment, or from abnormal bone growth such as in osteophyte formation.

The symptoms of low back pain include:

- Persistent pain in the lower back ranging from mild to excruciating, often incapacitating (many people with backache are unable to travel to their physician's office)
- Back feels as if it's "locked" and cannot move in certain positions

- Pain can be sudden, delayed, or gradual onset but usually with a history of a triggering event (usually a bending forward or twisting movement)
- Stiffness, especially after sitting for extended periods (most people with backache prefer to stand)
- Changes in posture and/or limitation of mobility and activity
- Often a history of previous episodes of back pain

The normal healing process can take from two to four weeks in 90 percent of people with backache, but the pain usually starts to decrease after a few days or a week.

Although backache is rarely life-threatening, the following types of back pain need the urgent attention of a physician. If you have any of these symptoms, have them evaluated as soon as possible.

- Sudden, severe back pain associated with pain in the abdominal area and shortness of breath, especially when there is no injury. This could be an aneurysm in the aorta (large blood vessel in the back).
- Weakness or inability to move your leg(s), with or without back pain, could be a stroke or a severe ruptured disc.
- Persistent back pain in one place could be a sign of bone disease or cancer. X rays or other tests may be helpful in making the diagnosis.

CAUSES AND RISK FACTORS OF BACKACHE

- Lifting heavy objects improperly, e.g., bending forward or moving too quickly or awkwardly
- Prolonged sitting, even with good posture, and a sedentary lifestyle are responsible for poorly conditioned muscles (both back and abdominal). The muscles become both weak and inflexible.
- Excessive exercise

- Emotional stress (refer to Chapter 5, page 205). Breath-holding, or shallow, rapid breathing that often occurs during times of stress, can stiffen and cause tension in the muscles of the spine. This not only contributes to compression forces in the spine, but can set the stage for even a minor physical incident, such as bending over, to throw the back out of balance and cause back pain.
- Poor posture and leg-length discrepancy
- Prolonged standing, insufficient arch support, and inappropriate footwear, such as high heels
- Obesity and pregnancy
- Inadequate support from a soft mattress
- Uncomfortable workstations, such as chairs with improper support or working under an automobile or with heavy equipment
- Nutritional deficiencies, especially low protein and magnesium intake (diuretics used to treat high blood pressure can lower magnesium)
- Constipation
- Congenital abnormalities of the spine predisposing to instability, such as a transitional articulated sixth lumbar vertebra

CONVENTIONAL MEDICAL TREATMENT OF BACKACHE

Most of the following therapies are helpful in providing temporary symptomatic relief for *acute* low back pain. Physical therapy, however, can be extremely effective for long-term improvement of chronic back pain (see page 33). Conventional therapies include:

(1) *Bedrest,* for no more than two days; and *limited activity*
(2) *Sleeping on the back* with a big pillow under the knees or on the side with a big pillow between the knees
(3) *Ice* to the affected area for the first two days. It can be applied hourly for 20 minutes at a time to help decrease swelling and pain.
(4) After two days, change to *moist heat* (heating pad, hot bath

or shower) to help loosen the muscles and decrease spasm. Begin gentle *stretching* to the point of tolerance (no pain). It is very important to listen to your body and not overstretch it. The intensity of the stretches may be very gradually increased daily until a return to full motion (or even better motion than originally) is attained. If you're not patient with this healing process, you may re-injure the muscle and have to start over. Refer to page 131 for stretching exercises.

(5) *Pain medications* are not curative and do not address the underlying causes of backache. They are preferred for acute back pain, not for management of chronic conditions. The most frequently recommended medications include: Tylenol, one to two extra-strength, 500 mg tablets, four times a day (maximum eight per day); aspirin, one to two tablets every four hours; ibuprofen (Advil, Nuprin, Motrin), 200 mg tablets, two to four tablets, three to four times a day; or naproxen sodium (Aleve), 220 mg, one tablet, two to three times a day. Even the newest nonsteroidal anti-inflammatories (NSAIDs), Celebrex and Vioxx, have been prescribed for treatment of back pain. However, they are of limited value since they do not address the muscular aspect of back pain. Tylenol has the fewest potential side effects of all the medications but may not provide as much pain relief. For short periods of time, all of these drugs are relatively safe. The exceptions are for persons with stomach ulcers or kidney and liver problems. None of them should be taken with alcohol, including the Tylenol. These medications can be purchased over the counter, or similar stronger versions can be prescribed by a physician, e.g., Celebrex and Vioxx. *Narcotic pain medications* are also used for short-term treatment of acute pain and can help for sleep as well. But they are highly addictive and should be used with great caution. There is also the risk of masking the pain to such an extent that you can re-injure your back and be unaware of it.

(6) *Muscle relaxants* may be prescribed if muscle spasm is a significant component of the back pain. These medications usually offer only moderate benefits at best and are not

meant for long-term use. They can be helpful to use at night for problems with sleep. The most commonly prescribed muscle relaxants are Flexeril, Norflex, Parafon Forte, Robaxin, and Soma. Most of them can cause drowsiness.

(7) *Antidepressants* may be helpful for treatment of chronic pain with accompanying depression. They increase levels of the neurotransmitter serotonin, which can reduce pain. They can also cause dizziness and drowsiness along with many other possible side effects.

(8) *Corticosteroids* act as anti-inflammatories and are usually injected into the epidural space. Relief can last for several months.

(9) *Physical therapy* is probably the *most effective conventional therapy in producing long-term benefits* for chronic low back pain. It is a multifaceted therapy that can address posture, the ergonomics of the workstation, and proper instruction in body mechanics—lifting and carrying (see page 144). Physical therapy includes a wide range of modalities, including traction, stretching, strength training, ultrasound, electrical stimulation, supervised exercises to improve range of motion, neuromuscular re-education, and therapeutic exercises. Physical therapists also administer work hardening programs and functional capacity exams to help with workmen's compensation cases to determine when the patient is ready to return to work. Many physical therapists also have training in sports medicine and in gentle complementary therapies such as yoga, tai chi, or Pilates.

(10) *Injections* of local anesthetics and saline into muscle trigger points frequently give temporary and sometimes long-lasting relief.

(11) *Surgery* should be considered as a last resort when all other options (including the therapies described in Chapter 4) have failed, since it's expensive (average cost is $35,000) and often doesn't produce long-term relief. It is most often performed for treatment of herniated discs (the procedure is called a *diskectomy,* often accompanied by a *laminectomy,* depending on the location of the herniation) and can be

initially helpful for pain relief. Statistics show that sciatica is relieved completely in 75 to 90 percent of patients and partially in another 15 percent. Back pain is eliminated in 70 percent of patients. Yet some studies are revealing *no difference in long-term improvement* (four years later) of back pain, whether surgery was performed or conservative management (such as bedrest and exercises) was used. Diskectomy leaves behind the weakened disc, which is less able to bear normal loads. This allows for continued deterioration of the adjacent vertebrae and recurrence of pain. *Spinal fusion,* often performed along with a diskectomy to stabilize the back, may also cause further degenerative changes. For these reasons, a growing number of medical researchers are working to develop a durable, effective, artificial disc that would not only provide the flexibility and load-carrying ability of a natural disc but also would prevent further degeneration by preserving the normal mechanics of the spine. Clinical trials are currently under way to determine the effectiveness of these devices.

Other less invasive surgical options include *microdiskectomy,* which is performed under magnification through a small (1-inch) opening; *arthroscopic percutaneous diskectomy,* which involves inserting a probe into the disc to scoop it out; *intradiskal electrothermoplaty,* in which a heated wire is inserted directly into the disc to burn it; and *laser diskectomy,* which uses a laser to burn out the disc. There are benefits and liabilities to each of these procedures, without any conclusive evidence that they produce any better long-term pain relief than the standard diskectomy. Another less invasive alternative to surgery is *chymopapain* treatment. Used far more frequently in Japan and Europe, it involves injecting chymopapain (an enzyme derived from papaya) into a herniated disc to dissolve it. Many American orthopedic surgeons and neurosurgeons are hesitant to use this treatment because of the 1 percent risk of an anaphylactic (severe allergic) reaction. It has a 70 percent efficacy rate in relieving pain.

The true indications for surgery include the following:

- A medical emergency or major injury, including unstable fractures
- Evidence of a spinal tumor
- Severe radiculopathy (pain radiating down leg) of one to three months with muscle atrophy in the affected leg
- Cauda equina syndrome—persistent groin and inner-thigh numbness, called "saddle anesthesia"; compromise of bowel or bladder function

(12) *Mechanical noninvasive therapies* (all are used for treating herniated discs) include:

- *Traction devices* work on the premise of decompressing the spine by increasing the space between the vertebrae to relieve pressure on the disc. They can be helpful in an acute setting.
- *Inversion systems* are self-administered traction, with the same therapeutic premise as above; they include hanging boots and related equipment.
- *VAX-D* (vertebral-axial decompression) is a relatively new stretching technique administered on a special table by a certified practitioner; five treatments per week for one month is recommended (average cost: $3,000); one study showed a 71 percent reduction in low back pain.
- *Chi machine,* a home-administered stretching and mild-traction device, may be effective for some people.

(13) *Spinal stenosis treatment* for those with mild cases and who are not candidates for surgery, then NSAIDs for pain, weight loss, and, especially, exercises to increase flexibility are recommended. Some success has been reported with the use of caudal epidural blocks—injections of analgesic drugs and a steroid directly into the base of the spine. Surgery is only considered when these measures fail to control symptoms or with impaired bladder or bowel function.

Chapter 3

HOLISTIC HEALTH: THE WELLNESS SELF-TEST

"The only thing I know that truly heals people is unconditional love."

ELISABETH KÜBLER-ROSS, M.D.

Most people who read this book probably have chronic low back pain and may not consider themselves to be particularly healthy. But *what is health?* The conditioning that the majority of us have grown up with has taught us to define "health" as the absence of illness. We may respond to the question "Are you healthy?" by thinking, *I'm not sick, so I must be healthy.* Yet the words "health," "heal," and "holy" are all derived from the same Old English word, *haelan,* which means "to make whole." Viewed from this perspective, two questions that more directly and accurately address the issue of health are, "Do you love your life?" or "Are you happy to be alive?" For health is far more than simply a matter of not feeling ill: It is the daily experience of *wholeness and balance—a state of being fully alive in body, mind, and spirit.* Such a condition could also be called optimal, or holistic, health or wellness. I call it *thriving.* Helping you to achieve this state of total well-being is the primary objective of this book. *As a by-product of that enlivening process, your backache will either improve significantly or be cured.*

HALLMARKS OF OPTIMAL HEALTH

Optimal health results from harmony and balance in the physical, environmental, mental, emotional, spiritual, and social aspects of our lives. When this harmonious balance is present, we experience the *unlimited and unimpeded free flow of life force energy throughout our body, mind, and spirit.* Around the world, this energy is known by many names. The Chinese call it *qi* ("chee"), the Japanese refer to it as *ki,* in India it is known as *prana,* and in Hebrew it is *chai.* But in the Western world, the term that comes closest to capturing the feeling generated by this energy is *unconditional love,* regarded by holistic physicians as *our most powerful healer.*

Although each of us has the capacity to nurture and to heal ourselves, most of us have yet to tap into this wellspring of loving life energy. Yet there is no one who can better administer this life-enhancing elixir to you than you yourself.

By committing to caring for yourself in the manner recommended in the following chapters, you will in essence be learning how to better *give and receive love*—to yourself and others. As a result, you will be enhancing the flow of life force energy throughout every aspect of your life. This holistic healing process will also provide you with the opportunity to safely and effectively treat your backache and any other physical, mental, and spiritual conditions that may be impeding the flow of healing energy in your life.

Living a holistically healthy lifestyle can facilitate the realization of your ideal life vision in accordance with both your personal and professional goals. But since the majority of us are only aware of health as a condition of not being sick, a mental image of what living holistically means is needed in order to achieve it. Briefly, let's examine this state of optimal well-being to give you a glimpse of what it looks and feels like.

A list of the six components of health follows, the first italicized item in each category encompassing the essence of that component. For example, physical health can be simply described as a condition of *high energy and vitality,* while mental health is a state of *peace of mind and contentment.* The italicized items can also serve as a health gauge that you can use to measure your progress in each area.

PHYSICAL HEALTH

High energy and vitality

- Freedom from, or high adaptability to, pain, dysfunction, and disability
- A strong immune system
- A body that feels light, balanced, strong, flexible, and has good aerobic capacity
- Ability to meet physical challenges and perform exceptionally
- Full capacity of all five senses and a healthy libido

ENVIRONMENTAL HEALTH

Harmony with your environment (neither harming nor being harmed)

- Awareness of your connectedness with nature
- Feeling grounded—comfort and security within your surroundings
- Respect and appreciation for your home, the Earth, and all of her inhabitants
- Contact with the earth; breathing healthy air; drinking pure water; eating uncontaminated food; exposure to the sun, fire, or candlelight; immersion in warm water (all on a daily basis)

MENTAL HEALTH

Peace of mind and contentment

- A job that you love doing
- Optimism
- A sense of humor
- Financial well-being
- Living your life vision
- The ability to express your creativity and talents
- The capacity to make healthy decisions

EMOTIONAL HEALTH

Self-acceptance and high self-esteem

- The capacity to identify, express, experience, and accept all of your feelings, both painful and joyful
- Awareness of the intimate connection between your physical and emotional bodies
- The ability to confront your greatest fears
- The fulfillment of your capacity to play
- Peak experiences on a regular basis

SPIRITUAL HEALTH

Experience of unconditional love/absence of fear

- Soul awareness and a personal relationship with God or Spirit
- Trusting your intuition and a willingness to change
- Gratitude
- Creating a sacred space on a regular basis through prayer, meditation, walking in nature, observing a Sabbath day, or other rituals
- Sense of purpose
- Being present in every moment

SOCIAL HEALTH

Intimacy with a spouse or partner, relative, or close friend

- Effective communication
- Forgiveness
- Touch and/or physical intimacy on a daily basis
- Recreation
- Sense of belonging to a support group or community
- Selflessness and altruism

THE WELLNESS SELF-TEST

Now that you understand the six categories that constitute optimal health, it's time to measure how close you are to *thriving* in each area. The following questionnaire is designed to provide you with a much clearer idea of the status of your health in all six areas. You can use the results of the test to guide you through the rest of the book, and it can become a blueprint for restructuring your life. You can also measure your progress by retaking the test every two or three months.

Answer the questions in each section below and total your score. Each response will be a number from 0 to 5. Please refer to the frequency described within the parentheses (e.g., "2 to 3 times/week") when answering questions about an *activity,* for example, "Do you maintain a healthy diet?" However, when the question refers to an *attitude* or an *emotion* (most of the *Mind and Spirit* questions, for example, "Do you have a sense of humor?"), the response is more subjective and less exact, and you should refer to the terms describing the frequency such as *often* or *daily,* but not to the numbered frequencies in parentheses.

0 = Never or almost never (once a year or less)
1 = Seldom (2 to 12 times/year)
2 = Occasionally (2 to 4 times/month)
3 = Often (2 to 3 times/week)
4 = Regularly (4 to 6 times/week)
5 = Daily (every day)

BODY: PHYSICAL AND ENVIRONMENTAL HEALTH

_____ 1. Do you maintain a healthy diet (low fat, low sugar, fresh fruits, grains, and vegetables)?

_____ 2. Is your water intake adequate (at least ½ oz/lb of body weight; 160 lbs = 80 ounces)?

_____ 3. Are you within 20 percent of your ideal body weight?

_____ 4. Do you feel physically attractive?

_____ 5. Do you fall asleep easily and sleep soundly?

_____ 6. Do you awaken in the morning feeling well rested?

_____ 7. Do you have more than enough energy to meet your daily responsibilities?

_____ 8. Are your five senses acute?

_____ 9. Do you take time to experience sensual pleasure?

_____10. Do you schedule regular massage or deep-tissue bodywork?

_____11. Does your sexual relationship feel gratifying?

_____12. Do you engage in regular physical workouts (lasting at least 20 minutes)?

_____13. Do you have good endurance or aerobic capacity?

_____14. Do you breathe abdominally for at least a few minutes?

_____15. Do you maintain physically challenging goals?

_____16. Are you physically strong?

_____17. Do you do some stretching exercises?

_____18. Are you free of chronic aches, pains, ailments, and diseases?

_____19. Do you have regular, effortless bowel movements?

_____20. Do you understand the causes of your chronic physical problems?

_____21. Are you free of any drug (including caffeine and nicotine) or alcohol dependency?

_____22. Do you live and work in a healthy environment with respect to clean air, water, and indoor pollution?

_____23. Do you feel energized or empowered by nature?

_____24. Do you feel a strong connection with and appreciation for your body, your home, and your environment?

_____25. Do you have an awareness of life force energy or *qi* ("chee")?

TOTAL BODY SCORE _____

MIND: MENTAL AND EMOTIONAL HEALTH

_____ 1. Do you have specific goals in your personal and professional life?

_____ 2. Do you have the ability to concentrate for extended periods of time?

_____ 3. Do you use visualization or mental imagery to help you attain your goals or enhance your performance?

_____ 4. Do you believe it is possible to change?

_____ 5. Can you meet your financial needs and desires?

_____ 6. Is your outlook basically optimistic?

_____ 7. Do you give yourself more supportive messages than critical messages?

_____ 8. Does your job utilize all of your greatest talents?

_____ 9. Is your job enjoyable and fulfilling?

_____10. Are you willing to take risks or make mistakes in order to succeed?

_____11. Are you able to adjust beliefs and attitudes as a result of learning from painful experiences?

_____12. Do you have a sense of humor?

_____13. Do you maintain peace of mind and tranquillity?

_____14. Are you free from a strong need for control or the need to be right?

_____15. Are you able to fully experience (feel) your painful feelings such as fear, anger, sadness, and hopelessness?

_____16. Are you aware of and able to safely express fear?

_____17. Are you aware of and able to safely express anger?

_____18. Are you aware of and able to safely express sadness (or cry)?

_____19. Are you accepting of all your feelings?

_____20. Do you engage in meditation, contemplation, or psychotherapy to better understand your feelings?

_____21. Is your sleep free from disturbing dreams?

_____22. Do you explore the symbolism and emotional content of your dreams?

_____23. Do you take the time to relax or make time for activities that constitute the abandon or absorption of play?

_____24. Do you experience feelings of exhilaration?

_____25. Do you enjoy high self-esteem?

TOTAL MIND SCORE _____

SPIRIT: SPIRITUAL AND SOCIAL HEALTH

_____ 1. Do you actively commit time to your spiritual life?

_____ 2. Do you take time for prayer, meditation, or reflection?

_____ 3. Do you listen to and act upon your intuition?

_____ 4. Are creative activities a part of your work or leisure time?

_____ 5. Do you take risks?

_____ 6. Do you have faith in a God, spirit guides, or angels?

_____ 7. Are you free from anger toward God?

_____ 8. Are you grateful for the blessings in your life?

_____ 9. Do you take walks, garden, or have contact with nature?

_____10. Are you able to let go of your attachment to specific outcomes and embrace uncertainty?

_____11. Do you observe a day of rest completely away from work, dedicated to nurturing yourself and your family?

_____12. Can you let go of self-interest in deciding the best course of action for a given situation?

_____13. Do you feel a sense of purpose?

_____14. Do you make time to connect with young children, either your own or someone else's?

_____15. Are playfulness and humor important to you in your daily life?

_____16. Do you have the ability to forgive yourself and others?

_____17. Have you demonstrated the willingness to commit to a marriage or comparable long-term relationship?

_____18. Do you experience intimacy, besides sex, in your committed relationships?

_____19. Do you confide in or speak openly with one or more close friends?

_____20. Do you or did you feel close to your parents?

_____21. If you have experienced the loss of a loved one, have you fully grieved that loss?

_____22. Has your experience of pain enabled you to grow spiritually?

_____23. Do you go out of your way or give your time to help others?

_____24. Do you feel a sense of belonging to a group or community?

_____25. Do you experience unconditional love?

TOTAL SPIRIT SCORE _____

TOTAL BODY, MIND, SPIRIT SCORE _____

HEALTH SCALE:

325–375	Optimal Health: *Thriving*
275–324	Excellent Health
225–274	Good Health
175–224	Fair Health
125–174	Below-Average Health
75–124	Poor Health
Less than 75	Extremely Unhealthy: *Surviving*

Once you complete this questionnaire, pay attention to which categories you need to make the most improvements in, and remember that *there are multiple factors that have combined to cause your back pain*. Then start to implement the tools and suggestions that are outlined in chapters 4, 5, and 6. Chapter 4 gives you a blueprint for improving your physical and environmental health while also specifically addressing backache; Chapter 5 outlines a holistic approach for mental and emotional health; while Chapter 6 will help you enhance your spiritual and social health. Begin where you are most comfortable and take your time. You are committing to a life-changing process, one that requires patience and discipline, so proceed at your own pace. Remember, too, that everyone is unique, and no two of us will follow the exact same healing path. While the science of holistic medicine provides a universal foundation and structure, its *art* lies in the writing of your own personal prescription for optimal health, so feel free to adapt the techniques in the pages ahead to tailor-make the holistic self-care program that is most ideally suited for you. Your heart will be your primary guide on this odyssey of realizing your full potential as a human being.

THE ESSENTIAL 8 FOR OPTIMAL HEALTH

During the fifteen years that I've been actively engaged in this healing process, I've identified several practices that have had the deepest impact on my health, the most transformative effect on my life, and will provide the greatest therapeutic benefits for your backache. I call them the *Essential 8 for Optimal Health*. These are:

(1) Air and breathing
(2) Water and moisture
(3) Food and supplements
(4) Exercise and rest
(5) Play/passion/purpose
(6) Gratitude/prayer/meditation

(7) Intimacy and connection

(8) Forgiveness

As you read the following chapters and begin incorporating the Backache Survival Program into your life, keep these Essential 8 in mind. (I've numbered them throughout the book, 1 through 8, to help you remember.) They are the basis of this holistic treatment program and can become the structure upon which the rest of your life is built.

Chapter 4

HEALING YOUR BODY:
The Physical and Environmental Health Components of the Backache Survival Program

I f you would rather not learn to live with your backache, along with its diminished quality of life, then I would like to take you on a healing journey into an exciting new (yet ancient) frontier of medicine. For the past fifteen years, I have been practicing *holistic medicine* while treating backache, arthritis, sinusitis, headache, and a variety of other so-called chronic or "incurable" conditions. The Backache Survival Program has its foundation in the holistic medical practice of treating, preventing, and potentially curing any chronic condition, as well as creating a state of optimal well-being. Although the bulk of the holistic approach is similar for any chronic condition or disease, this chapter and those that follow include specific exercises; dietary, nutritional supplement, and herbal recommendations; professional care therapies; as well as emotional factors that directly relate to treating the causes and symptoms of backache. They can be used as an alternative or a complement to the conventional medical treatment, such as medication or physical therapy, that you might already be doing. Holistic medicine can also be an excellent means of strengthening your low back following surgery and a highly effective method of preventing recurrence of backache in the event that your conventional treatment has been successful. This is not an "either/or" situation where you must choose one or the other. Holistic medicine is inclusive of conventional therapies. It is *not* alternative medicine. The intent is to use whatever is safe and effective in treating chronic ailments.

Commitment to the holistic approach has resulted in a significant improvement or elimination of back pain, in addition to a far greater experience of well-being in many people. This success stems primarily from the basic *health orientation* of the holistic approach. Rather than focusing on the physical condition and just treating its symptoms—they are certainly not ignored, just perceived differently—holistic medicine addresses *causes* while restoring balance and harmony to the *whole person*. It goes far beyond the "quick fix" or the repair of a "broken part," to an understanding of what can be learned from your physical pain and how to use that knowledge to take better care of yourself, change your life, and be free of back pain.

I was led to the practice of holistic medicine and a condition of optimal health by my painful sinuses. My guide on this healing path was, and still is, Hippocrates, who recognized 2,500 years ago the most direct and effective method for training to become a healer: "Physician heal thyself." In the remainder of this book, I'd like to guide you on a similar path, leading not only to the healing of your backache and any other dis-ease but also to a state of holistic health. By taking the Wellness Self-Test contained in Chapter 3, you have measured your present state of well-being. I'd recommend repeating this test every two to three months to gauge your physical, environmental, mental, emotional, spiritual, and social health progress and your training as *a healer of yourself*.

In the process of healing your body along with your painful back, the ultimate objectives are the following state of physical and environmental well-being.

COMPONENTS OF PHYSICAL HEALTH

High energy and vitality

- Freedom from, or high adaptability to, pain, dysfunction, and disability

- A strong immune system
- A body that feels light, balanced, strong, flexible, and has good aerobic capacity
- Ability to meet physical challenges and perform exceptionally
- Full capacity of all five senses and a healthy libido

COMPONENTS OF OPTIMAL ENVIRONMENTAL HEALTH

Harmony with your environment (neither harming nor being harmed)

- Awareness of your connectedness with nature
- Feeling grounded—comfort and security within your surroundings
- Respect and appreciation for your home, the Earth, and all of her inhabitants
- Contact with the earth; breathing healthy air; drinking pure water; eating uncontaminated food; exposure to the sun, fire, or candlelight; immersion in warm water (all on a daily basis)

HOLISTIC MEDICAL TREATMENT AND PREVENTION

To begin to restore your body to a heightened state of harmony and to correct the present imbalance manifested by back pain, your *primary goals* are:

- To relax the muscles and relieve inflammation in your low back
- To enhance blood flow and strengthen the tissues of your low back
- To address each of the possible causes of your backache

In meeting these goals you can potentially cure your chronic low back pain while you're healing your life. The word "cure" refers to a physical problem, while "heal" has to do with the condition of your life. It is, however, possible to cure your backache but still be living an imbalanced life; or conversely, you may feel whole, balanced, and at peace with your life while still experiencing some degree of back pain. In essence, *this holistic approach will provide you with the potential to do both—cure backache and heal your life—while you are engaged in the process of loving and nurturing your pained, contracted, and inflamed low back along with the rest of you.* As you begin, you should now keep in mind the image of yourself as completely relaxed, highly flexible, and pain-free. You see yourself bending forward and placing your palms on the floor, then bending backward and touching the floor with all of your fingers while forming a "body bridge." Your body looks and feels vibrantly healthy, supple, and strong. This healing vision can be expanded in any way you'd like. But it is important to keep it in mind as often as you can, since it will help you to stay focused on the goal of your treatment and, even more important, to make that *vision become a reality.*

Think of the Backache Survival Program as a *personalized course in self-healing and optimal well-being.* In this and the following chapters, you will be provided with a "curriculum" or, if you prefer, a "prescription," for improving the six components of health, while treating each of the primary causes of backache. I have tried to simplify each component and have suggested "exercises" to help you find your own path to a greater level of physical, environmental, mental, emotional, spiritual, and social fitness. These exercises must be practiced regularly in order to be effective. (However, if after giving it a fair trial, a particular exercise feels too uncomfortable to you, then stop.) If you are willing to be patient—remember, it took years for you to develop your current state of health—I promise that you will feel better, but I cannot guarantee that you will be cured of back pain. However, your chances for doing so are far greater using this approach, especially if there is no major disc degeneration or spinal stenosis, than if you strictly adhered to the conventional medical treatment that treats only symptoms. As a complement to what you are already doing for your backache, holistic medicine is the most therapeutically sound and cost-effective approach to the treatment of chronic disease that I've found in over thirty years of practicing medicine. By taking responsibility for your own health, you become not only your own healer but also a highly skilled practitioner of preventive medicine. You will learn what *causes* your back to ache and what relieves the pain, and will be able to make well-informed choices regarding your treatment of this condition. You're also somewhat of a pioneer, since the holistic self-care model presented on the following pages will soon become an essential part of the foundation of primary care medicine. Keep in mind that although this is a course with a lot of homework, there are no exams or grades, no mistakes or failures, just a series of valuable lessons to help you feel more fully alive. Enjoy yourself! What do you have to lose?

The foundation of the physical aspect of the holistic medical treatment is to love and nurture your body with safe, gentle, and effective therapies. You should have a much better idea of how to do that, especially for your aching back, after reading this chapter. Remember that the "quick-fix" essentials of the physical health components of the Backache Survival Program can also be found in Chapter 1.

SYMPTOM TREATMENT

I would recommend beginning the Backache Survival Program with an aggressive approach to treating your symptoms while attempting to identify their causes. This includes consulting with your physician and making sure that you have treated your condition with the best methods that conventional medicine has to offer, even if they provide only temporary and symptomatic relief. It is also essential that you determine if the benefits of that treatment outweigh the liabilities. For instance, analgesics and anti-inflammatories may be harmful to the gastrointestinal tract, possibly causing stomach ulcers. Muscle relaxants might make you feel drowsy or a bit spacey. If you've decided the risks for continuing this course of symptom treatment are too great or that it's not giving you effective relief, there are a multitude of options that will be offered to you in this chapter.

As you begin the Backache Survival Program, it is helpful to rate each of your symptoms on a scale of 1 to 10, with 1 being an almost incapacitating symptom and 10 being perfectly normal (no symptom). You can use the "Symptom Chart" (pages 52 and 53) and rate yourself at the end of each week. It provides you with both an objective (most of the symptoms can be measured objectively—you can either see, hear, or feel them) and a subjective (energy level, emotions) means of monitoring your progress. At the same time, you are also paying close attention to your stress level, activities, diet, and any other factor you suspect may be triggering your back pain. In evaluating your own symptoms, you don't need anyone else or an X ray or lab test to tell you how well you're doing. Please add any symptoms to this chart that are not listed but that often cause you discomfort. You can modify this chart in whatever way you'd like. Be creative with it. You can add a section for activities, more space for additional emotions, and whatever else you think might be contributing to your backache.

PHYSICAL AND ENVIRONMENTAL HEALTH RECOMMENDATIONS FOR BACKACHE

Backache, like any other chronic condition viewed from a holistic medical perspective, is a systemic dis-ease reflecting an imbalance and disharmony in the whole person—body, mind, and spirit. However, if your initial treatment is aggressively directed toward healing and restoring balance to the low back, and subsequently your mental and spiritual health, and there is no major disc degeneration or spinal stenosis, you have an excellent chance of curing your backache using this holistic approach.

The primary goals of treatment are to *relax the muscles, relieve inflammation, enhance blood flow, and strengthen the tissues of your low back.* In holistic medicine, this objective equates to the physical response to nurturing the painful back. Physiologically, every organ, tissue, and body part functions more efficiently with a maximal supply of oxygen—our body's most critical nutrient—

Symptom Chart

Began Backache Survival Program on _____
Rate symptoms from 1 (worst) to 10 (best = normal)

SYMPTOM	BEGIN ___ (date)	END WEEK 1	END WEEK 2	END WEEK 3	END WEEK 4	END WEEK 5	END WEEK 6	END WEEK 7	END WEEK 8	END WEEK 9	END WEEK 10	END WEEK 11	END WEEK 12
Pain													
Immobility (getting out of bed or out of a chair)													
Stiffness (ability to bend or twist)													
Radiating pain (into your leg or buttock)													
Numbness or tingling													
Energy level/ stamina													
Sleep quality													
Irritability													
Depression													
Anxiety/worry													
Other symptoms:													

SYMPTOM	BEGIN ____ (date)	END WEEK 1	END WEEK 2	END WEEK 3	END WEEK 4	END WEEK 5	END WEEK 6	END WEEK 7	END WEEK 8	END WEEK 9	END WEEK 10	END WEEK 11	END WEEK 12
Medications: (pharmaceutical drugs) (use a "√" if still taking drug)													
Vitamins/herbs/ supplements (use a "√" if still taking)													

along with the other essential nutrients. Since oxygen and all nutrients are transported through the blood, and blood consists almost entirely of water, anything that *enhances blood flow* to the low back should relieve the condition. This might include increased water intake, breathing exercises and meditation, yoga and stretching, massage and bodywork, exercise, healing touch, and physical therapy. Reducing stress on the back, such as losing weight, improving workplace ergonomics, reducing activity, and eliminating any foods or other triggers of inflammation if arthritis or a degenerative disc is responsible for the back pain, are also methods of directly relieving pain.

Throughout the remainder of this chapter, I will incorporate the most effective physical methods for healing backache into the Essential 8 for Optimal Health that I listed at the conclusion of Chapter 3. This will allow you to feel much healthier than you may ever have before while you're in the process of healing your aching back. The eight health practices will be numbered in the same way as before, and this chapter will include numbers 1 through 4. We'll begin with item 1—Air and Breathing.

1. AIR AND BREATHING

There is nothing more important to optimal health and survival than the quality of the air and our ability to breathe it. The more efficiently we breathe, the more oxygen we inhale, and the greater the potential to relax and strengthen the muscles and tissues of the low back, along with every other part of the body. There are several environmental factors that can result in a lack of oxygen, such as air pollution, high altitude, and carbon monoxide. It is also possible to experience an oxygen deficiency from breathing inefficiently or if the nose and sinuses are not functioning at peak efficiency—they might be congested or infected with allergies, a cold, or a sinus infection. In the following pages I will describe how to create optimal indoor air and recommend several exercises for more efficient breathing.

OPTIMAL AIR QUALITY

The first step in improving both your physical and environmental health is to change the quality of the indoor air you're breathing—in essence, to create healing, rather than harmful or irritating, air. All of the recommendations mentioned in this section are helpful. But, at the very least, I would start with a negative-ion generator in your bedroom and, if you can afford it, in your workplace as well. I would then add a warm-mist humidifier in the bedroom (especially during the winter months), along with plants in the house, an effective furnace filter, followed by air duct and carpet cleaning. If the expense does not deter you, then a central humidifier installed on the furnace will complete your indoor air-enhancement program. You may not create optimal indoor air, but you'll be close.

Ideal air quality is rated by clarity (freedom from pollutants), humidity (between 35 and 55 percent), temperature (between 65° and 85°F), oxygen content (21 percent of total volume and 100 percent saturation), and negative-ion content (3,000 to 6,000 .001-micron ions per cubic centimeter). Air that is clean, moist, warm, oxygen-rich, and high in negative ions is the healthiest air a human being can breathe.

Not only are we dependent on oxygen for survival, but every part of the human body thrives with a maximum supply of oxygen. If your respiratory tract is defective because of a nasal, sinus, or lung ailment, or if the amount of oxygen available in the air is relatively low—air that is high in carbon monoxide and/or other pollutants, air at higher altitudes (oxygen content decreases by over 3 percent every thousand feet above sea level), or stale indoor air—your body is receiving less than its optimal requirement of oxygen. Headache is often the first symptom of a lack of oxygen. Scientists report that the oxygen content of the air in some polluted cities is as low as 8 percent instead of the normal 21 percent. If you live in a polluted high-altitude city such as Denver, Salt Lake City, or Albuquerque, then your body is receiving far less oxygen than it needs for optimal function. And if the muscles in your low back are tight, contracted, and constricting blood flow, then this area will receive even less oxygen. Tissues that are starved for oxygen typically respond with pain. Although headache is usually considered to be the earliest symptom of oxygen deprivation, backache may result from a very similar pathophysiologic process.

Negative ions are air molecules that have excess electrons. Negative ions vitalize or freshen the air we breathe by removing unhealthy particles. The Earth itself is a natural negative-ion generator. Health spas have always been located in areas high in negative ions (3,000 to 20,000 per cubic centimeter of air), such as along seacoasts, near rushing streams and waterfalls, in mountainous areas, and in pine forests (pine needles cause negative ions to be generated in the surrounding air). Although unproven, there is speculation that negative ions increase the sweeping motion of the cilia on the respiratory mucosa and subsequently enhance the movement of mucus and the clearing or filtering of inhaled pollutants. Unfortunately, there is very little research on the effect of negative ions on the respiratory tract. Two studies performed in the 1960s in Israel indicated that negative ions had a beneficial effect on asthmatics, but to my knowledge there has been no recent research.

However, what has been conclusively proven is that negative ions are effective air cleaners. They do so by attracting dust, smoke, mold, pollen, bacteria, and viruses, all of which have a positive charge. The heavier combined particle (the negative ion plus the pollutant) then falls from the air to the ground and is removed from the breathing space. Negative ions also have been shown to help reduce pain, heal burns, suppress mold and bacterial growth, stimulate plant growth, and contribute greatly to our sense of well-being and comfort.

Positive ions are air molecules lacking electrons. Pollen can carry fifty or more positive charges per grain of pollen. This positive charge slows the cilia and the clearing of mucus and in so doing can cause some degree of nasal congestion. Most man-made pollutants result from combustion processes (auto and truck exhaust, smokestacks, cigarette smoke, and the like) that leave the pollutants with a positive charge. Heating and ventilation systems tend to produce air containing an excess of positive ions. Aircraft cabins have been tested and found to contain an excessively high amount of positive ions. This obviously contributes to the "stuffy" feeling of airplane air and also helps to explain why so many of my patients have developed colds and sinus infections following air travel. Television and especially computer screens also emit an excess of positive ions, which draws negative ions out of the air and neutralizes them. This may contribute (along with poor posture) to the frequent backaches experienced by people spending extended periods of time operating a computer.

The negative-ion content of indoor air can be as low as 10 to 200 negative ions per cubic centimeter. This is considered to be "ion-depleted" air and is a significant component of "sick-building syndrome." Ion-depleted air is also created by heating/cooling systems, window air conditioners, and even air cleaners (including HEPA filters), which "scrub" negative ions from the air. Most of the factors in our environment responsible for depleting the beneficial negative ions also produce an excess of unhealthy positive ions.

The majority of Americans spend 90 percent of their time indoors, where, the EPA says, the air can be much more polluted than outdoor air. Few of us live in clean, moist environments that are warm year-round; even fewer live in the mountains, on a beach, or in the woods. For the 92 million people whose lungs, sinuses, and noses are already adversely affected from breathing unhealthy air, for the backache sufferer, and for anyone else who wants to enjoy optimum health, here are some ways to minimize the risks of breathing poor-quality air and to contribute toward the prevention of almost any chronic ailment.

Healthy Homes

Where we live, work, play, or otherwise spend our time is critical to our health. If you are considering a move, you should look for a home in a location that minimizes the impact of outdoor air pollution or in a city or town that has minimal air pollution. If you are going to relocate and have the freedom to choose, avoid the following regions: Southern California, the Northeast, and the Texas Gulf Coast. The healthiest air can be found along the West Coast (with the distinct exception of the Los Angeles metropolitan area and southward), rural areas along the Gulf Coast (other than Texas), and the west coast of Florida.

If you are contemplating the construction of a new home, the concept of *ecological architecture* could help considerably in creating a healthy environment. "Ecology" is defined in Webster's *New World Dictionary* as "the branch of biology that deals with the relationship between living organisms and their environment." Used as a modifier for the word "architecture," it simply means the design of a dwelling that is sensitive to human health and gentle to the Earth. Once we have considered the microclimate and the site, our biological needs, behavior patterns, and, most important, our budgetary limitations, nature will then dictate the design. Self-sufficiency through use of sun, air, earth, and water for heating, cooling, ventilation, and even electrical power is a realistic goal of an ecological design.

Common objectives regarding construction methods and materials include:

- Avoiding the use of plastic or other materials made of toxic ingredients that harmfully outgas (give off toxins and/or fumes) in the indoor environment
- Using nontoxic natural materials in preference to synthetic materials
- Designing with concern for sensitivities, allergies, or chronic health problems
- Being aware that nature's ecologic sustainability and well-being should not be diminished by what is built
- Taking the responsibility to conceive, design, build, and furnish a home or building to a "healthy home" ecological ethic

This is a holistic approach emphasizing the ecological bond between site and architecture. Preservation and wise use of our planet's resources in construction and throughout the lifetime of a home are fundamental to ecological design. Ideally, a home must be clean, moist, warm, and oxygen and negative-ion rich. The fact that it is designed in harmony with the atmosphere and the Earth makes this an environmentally healthy concept.

I fully appreciate that most readers of this book will neither move nor design their own homes as a result of what they read here. However, I want to present as many environmental treatment options as possible. Each can potentially have an indirect benefit to your backaches while also having a profound impact on your overall state of health and ultimately your quality of life. Fortunately, technology has made it possible to create an oasis of healthy indoor air in your own home, so you won't have to move or build a new home. In the desert, an oasis provides water. In the sea of hazardous air in which we live, a *healthy home or business* can provide an oasis in which to breathe life-enhancing air.

Solving the problem of indoor air pollution entails both treatment and prevention. There is a company in Denver, Healthy Habitats, that has been on the leading edge of this field for over fifteen years. The owner of the company, Carl Grimes, has worked with me and a number of my patients to transform our unhealthy homes and offices into healthy ones. The procedures and techniques he employs adhere to the following guidelines:

- Prevention—avoid bringing pollutants into the home and workplace
- Identify the source and develop a plan for isolating or removing the pollutant from the "breathing zone," or the surrounding area from which you obtain your breathing air—for example, an infant's breathing zone includes the floor and carpeting
- Reduce ambient pollution with ventilation, filtration, and ionization

Grimes considers the three primary sources of pollution to be:

- Particulates—dust, pollen, dander, construction debris, and smoke
- Microorganisms—bacteria, viruses, molds, and dust mites

• Chemicals and gases— personal care products, cleaning products, office equipment, and building/construction materials. (See Table 4.1 below.)

The type of treatment depends upon the type of pollution. For example, HEPA (high efficiency particulate arrestor) filtration might be used for particulates, charcoal for chemicals and

---

Table 4.1

Indoor Air Pollutants

Automotive Fumes
From outdoor traffic, outdoor parking lots, and outdoor loading and unloading spaces, as well as indoor garages

Chemicals and Chemical Solutions (Chemicals that affect indoor air quality are those associated with architecture, the interior, artifacts, and maintenance.)
Fungicides and pesticides in carpet-cleaning residues and sprays; formaldehyde, used in the manufacture of insulation, plywood, fiberboard, furniture, and wood paneling; toxic solvents in oil-based paints, finishes, and wall sealants; aerosol sprays; office equipment chemicals, especially photocopiers and computers

Combustion Products
Tobacco smoke★
Coal- or wood-burning fireplaces and stoves
Fuel combustion gases from gas-fired appliances such as ranges, clothes dryers, water heaters, and fireplaces (they produce nitrogen dioxide, carbon monoxide, nitrous oxides, sulfur oxides, hydrocarbons, and formaldehyde)

Ion Depletion or Imbalance
Too few negative ions
Excess of positive ions over negative ions

★From all of the available scientific data, tobacco smoke is the most unhealthy indoor air pollutant.

Microorganisms (primarily from humidifiers, air conditioners, and
any other building components affected by excessive moisture)
Bacteria
Viruses
Molds
Dust mites (usually found in more humid areas)

Particulates
Dust
Pollen
Animal dander
Particles (frayed materials)
Asbestos

Radionuclides
Radon, a radioactive gas emitted from the earth that enters homes
primarily through basements, crawl spaces, and water supply, especially from wells (it can attach to the particulates of cigarette
smoke, dust particles, and natural aerosols)

gases, and the drying of a wet crawl space could be the best option for eliminating microbes. Ozone has also been effective for
persistent microorganisms; however, when a home is cleaned
with ozone, the residents are advised to vacate the premises for
two to three days. Chemical and gaseous pollution is harder to
avoid than particulate matter. Although activated charcoal filters
may be effective for removing toxic gases (formaldehyde is the
most common gas found in homes), a simpler strategy involves
the use of house plants known to absorb gases from the air (see
page 70).

Molds are rapidly becoming one of America's chief health
hazards and are recognized as one of the leading causes for the
dramatic increase in asthma, allergies, and chronic sinusitis during the past twenty years. The reason many of us are being exposed daily to high levels of mold is primarily a result of modern
home design—more airtight, with air-conditioning and heating

systems recirculating contaminated air; materials used; and, most important, *water leaks.* Molds can grow wherever it's damp, so it's important to quickly fix any leaks, regularly clean air ducts and furnace filters, be on the lookout for discoloration of walls or ceilings and any unusual odors, and empty (daily) and clean (weekly) humidifiers on a regular basis.

Several excellent books are available on the subject of healthy homes. Those that I recommend are *Starting Points for a Healthy Habitat* by Carl Grimes (GMC Media); *The Nontoxic Home and Office* by Debra Lynn Dadd (Jeremy P. Tarcher, Inc.); *The Healthy House* by John Bower (Lyle Stuart, Inc.); and *Your Home, Your Health and Well-Being* by David Rousseau (Ten Speed Press).

Air Cleaners and Negative-Ion Generators

As many as 1 million hospital admissions a year are attributed to poor indoor air quality. In recent years, as the EPA and private health organizations have publicized the problem of indoor air pollution, we have seen a proliferation of several hundred types of air cleaners, almost as many as there are indoor air pollutants. According to Michael Berry, Ph.D., former manager of the EPA's Indoor Air Project, the most potentially harmful pollutants are radon and the "biologicals," including pollen, molds, plant spores, dust mites, bacteria, and viruses. The pollutants most harmful to the respiratory tract are less than one micron in size. Regardless of their origin, size, or health-damaging effects, air pollutants can be described as free-floating particles in the air.

Figure 4.1 shows the specific size ranges of the most common pollutants. The unit of measurement used for tiny air particles is the micron. An average hair strand is 100 microns thick, and about 400 one-micron particles would fit into the dot over the "i" in the word "micron." The primary job of air cleaners is to remove as many of these particles as possible, the biologicals as well as the combustion products, particulates, chemicals, fumes, and odors. Radon, if present, requires sealing basement cracks and improving basement ventilation. Most air cleaners do not

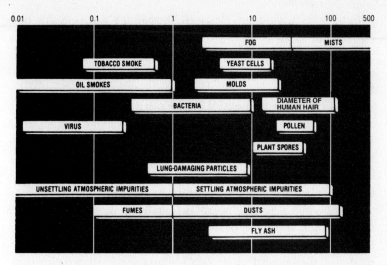

FIGURE 4.1   *Relative Size of Common Air Contaminants*

remove radon from the air. However, some air cleaners with high-particle removal efficiency (HEPA, for example) can remove some of the radon "daughters" (attached radon) that are in particulate form. A study at the Harvard School of Public Health determined that a negative-ion generator is a highly effective means of removing the attached fraction of radon (the radon daughters), although it does not reduce the unattached (gaseous) fraction of radon.

The strategy for solving the problem of indoor air pollution involves *air cleaning* and *improved ventilation*. Air-cleaning devices can include furnace filters, portable stand-alone units, and negative-ion generators. The efficiency of air cleaners is evaluated by their ability to filter a certain percentage of a certain size of pollutant. The HEPA filter removes 97 percent of all 0.3-micron particulates and larger. This includes pollen, mold, plant spores, most animal dander, dust, wood and tobacco smoke, fumes, bacteria, and some viruses. This type of filter is standard equipment for most hospital operating suites and is found in many of the more expensive freestanding air cleaners. It requires a strong fan or a booster fan to move air through it due to its increased efficiency.

The ULPA (ultra low penetrating air) filters were originally created to purify the air in semiconductor clean rooms. The Bionaire company has now made this new technology available to clean the air in homes. ULPA air purifiers are equipped with a superfine filter that removes a remarkable 99.999 percent of all airborne particles as small as 0.1 micron. The filter traps such allergens as tobacco smoke, pollen, dust, dust mites, mold, and bacteria. For best performance, it is recommended that ULPA filters be changed every six months to one year.

Negative-ion generators were originally designed to restore a more natural and beneficial level of negative ions to indoor air. In the course of their use for biological benefit, it was discovered that free-floating ions quickly attach to airborne particles and cause them to agglomerate and precipitate from the air, or be drawn to grounded surfaces such as walls and metal surfaces. Ionizers are highly effective air cleaners, removing particles as small as .001 micron, which would include viruses, molds, dust, pollen, cigarette smoke, and all other airborne particulate pollutants. Compared to air cleaners with fans or blowers, ionizers are more likely to be operated full-time since they are totally silent (no fan) and consume only pennies of electricity per month.

However, in order to increase the speed with which an ionizer cleans the air, many manufacturers produce ionizers with excessive ion output. This has two undesirable effects:

(1) The ion density established by these ionizers exceeds many times the natural range found outdoors, resulting in much the same adverse effects as breathing air with too few negative ions. A well-designed negative-ion generator will generate enough ions to be effective but will not exceed an upper limit that would make it biologically undesirable.

(2) An excessively high ion density also causes a significant amount of pollutants to be driven to the walls and other grounded surfaces, resulting in the buildup of a dirty residue.

Again, a well-designed ion generator will minimize such "plating," and this effect can be further reduced by placing the ionizer at least two feet from the nearest wall.

It has been my good fortune, and that of my patients, to have worked with a "pioneer" in negative-ion technology. For nearly thirty years, Rex Coppom, owner of Electrofilter Technologies in Longmont, Colorado, has been developing state-of-the-art negative-ion generators. For almost ten years, many of my patients have been using his Sinus Survival Air Vitalizer, a small unit that will clean the air of a 150- to 200-square-foot room. And its self-regulation feature enables it to maintain an ideal level of negative ions (3,000 to 6,000 per cubic centimeter). It costs $150, considerably less than the average price of a HEPA room air cleaner, which is somewhat less efficient in its cleaning capacity and has no negative ions. I have received many testimonials about its beneficial effects—dramatic headache relief, fewer allergy and asthma attacks, diminished nasal congestion, cessation of snoring, better sleep, more energy, general feelings of well-being, and diminished odor and symptoms resulting from secondhand cigarette smoke. I was amazed at how quickly it cleared the smoke from my kitchen during an oven-cleaning session that went somewhat awry. Ionization equipment is currently available for automobiles and aircraft cabins—both of which have far less than optimum air.

Electronic air cleaners (both central and freestanding) produce positive ions as they filter the air. On their first day of operation, they are 85 percent efficient on all 1-micron particles and larger; but in order to maintain that efficiency, they require cleaning every two weeks. For most of us, this makes them impractical and inconvenient. They also produce ozone, which can be a potential health hazard.

To obtain a *furnace filter,* go to a hardware or building-supply store. Many of them carry the 3M pleated filter, under the brand name Filtrete. These are excellent furnace filters and cost about $15. They should be replaced every one to two months during the winter and while central air conditioners are being run regularly. They are far more efficient than the $2 to $4 varieties found in supermarkets. There are several other brands of pleated furnace filters that are similar in efficiency to 3M.

The DuPont Wizard Dust Cloth is an interesting product that does a better job of dusting than can be obtained from liquid or spray dust cleaners. They are used dry, can be washed, and cost $2.

Air Duct Cleaning

When the air duct system of my thirteen-year-old home was cleaned for the first time, I was amazed at what emanated from the ducts after two hours of high-intensity vacuuming. I thought to myself, "It's no wonder I suffered with sinus problems for so long!" If the air ducts are filthy, it is nearly impossible for your furnace filter to clean the air in your home. After the air is filtered, it still has to travel through the ducts before you breathe it. I recommend air duct cleaning as part of the environmental treatment program. Depending on the size of your home, an air duct cleaning service, using good equipment, could cost between $200 and $250. To find this type of company in your city, look in the Yellow Pages under "Furnaces, Cleaning and Repairing."

Carpet Cleaning

Carpets are one of the most common sources of indoor air pollutants. They are excellent traps and hold on to dust, pollen, and microorganisms. While this helps to keep those particles out of the breathing zone, their gradual accumulation can become great enough to create a sustainable culture of bacteria, yeast, dust mites, and mold. In fact, many allergists recommend that their patients dispose of all their carpets.

While it is true that carpets harbor pollutants, it is possible to keep them clean. This poses a challenge to the homemaker. Conventional vacuum cleaners are designed to remove and retain the visible dirt, which means particles greater than 10 microns. Most of the particles and microorganisms that are too small to be seen are also smaller than the pores in the vacuum cleaner bag. This allows most of them to blow through the bag and into the room, settling back onto the carpets and furniture. If a forced-air heating system is running, the airborne particles can be drawn into the air ducts, contributing to their contamination as well. Also, as the bag fills, airflow decreases, causing uneven cleaning.

To prevent these problems, I suggest a vacuum cleaner that uses either a HEPA-type filter or water-capture. Either one can remove subvisible dust and bacteria from the air. The water-capture types also have a continuously maximum airflow because they won't clog like a bag or filter. Both of these vacuums are expensive, costing between $500 and $1,000.

However, there is a much less expensive alternative. Dupont Hysurf vacuum cleaner bags have 1-micron pores and cost only $5. They appear to have the equivalent cleaning efficiency of the $500-plus "allergy" vacuum cleaners. Their major problem is that they are difficult to find. Some janitorial supply houses and medical supply stores have them. They can also be obtained from Sinus Survival Services.

Many people have their carpets professionally cleaned. However, due to their chemical composition, the most common cleaning agents are often worse than having dirty carpets. Alcohols, petroleum distillates, ammonia, dry-cleaning substances, and scents often cause headaches, mental "fuzziness," lethargy, and a general feeling of discomfort. Cleaning-agent residues may often cause respiratory irritation.

Before contracting with a carpet cleaner, check his references and insist on a nonscented cleaning agent that uses no petroleum distillates, alcohol, ammonia, dry-cleaning–type chemicals or enzymes and has no suds that can be left in the carpet. Check his work to be sure he leaves no damp areas. This ensures maximum removal of all agents and enhances drying time. If the carpet stays wet for several days, bacteria and molds can grow rapidly.

Ventilation and Plants

All indoor spaces, whether residential, commercial, industrial, or recreational, require some type of ventilation to provide breathable air for occupants, to furnish combustion air for cooking and heating, and to remove stale air filled with toxins and particulates. Commercial buildings are required by code to have even more efficient ventilation systems than residences. The American Society of Heating, Refrigerating and Air-Conditioning Engineers (ASHRAE) says that air should be replaced at the rate of 15 cubic feet per minute per person, but most systems fall below this minimum standard.

Improving ventilation will help relieve indoor air pollution as long as the outdoor air isn't dirtier than the air it is replacing. Local pollution sources, such as fumes from toxic waste leakage, wood burning, a neighboring industrial plant, a heavily trafficked highway, or crop spraying can render outdoor air unacceptable for indoor ventilation. Several days a year, Los Angeles residents are advised to keep all windows and doors closed and ventilation ducts shut to prevent the heavily polluted outdoor air from entering homes and businesses. In areas like this, it becomes a challenge to balance the health benefit of highly oxygenated outdoor air and the liability of the pollutants that come with it. Outdoor aerobic exercise presents a similar dilemma. If you live in a heavily polluted environment, I recommend exercising outside and ventilating your home and office well when outdoor air is good, but exercise indoors and keep windows and doors closed during periods of heavy pollution.

Air-conditioning systems are a helpful means of ventilation for people with respiratory and allergy problems. These systems remove excess moisture from the air, lowering its temperature. In less humid conditions, there is a reduction of molds and spores; and with the windows closed, there is also a marked decrease in pollutants and pollen from the outdoors. Air conditioning, however, does deplete negative ions from the air.

Natural cross-ventilation is effective in reducing indoor air pollution if the placement of the intake vents is low and the outlets for the flow-through air are high. Operable windows on commercial buildings and a good location for the outdoor air intake—away from garage entrances or loading docks—are also important factors in improving indoor air quality. Mechanical ventilation with exhaust fans can certainly help in removing indoor pollutants, but such fans are most efficient when used in a confined space. Private offices or single-occupant rooms where smoking, cooking, and other fume-producing activities take place are ideal environments for mechanical ventilation.

Rooms producing commercial toxic or odoriferous fumes; spaces subject to bacterial and viral contamination, such as rest rooms; and indoor areas that present specific respiratory hazards all need optimized ventilation. Mold is a special problem in moist conditions. Adequate ventilation along with sunshine can help to reduce moisture and subsequently suppress mold.

The technology of ventilation can be complex, but the basic principle of displacing interior air with outdoor air and increasing the rate of fresh airflow is critical to treating the problem of indoor air pollution. Besides natural cross-ventilation and exhaust fans, other devices used to enhance ventilation and indoor air quality are air-to-air heat exchangers, makeup air units, attic fans, vortex fans, and ceiling fans. Remember that even if the "fresh" air is filthy, an effective air cleaner combined with good ventilation is still a winning combination.

Adequate ventilation not only helps reduce indoor air pollution but is the primary source of indoor oxygen. Plants can offer an aesthetically pleasant secondary source in addition to their ability to remove toxic gases from the air. *Plants can help improve indoor air as oxygenators, filters, and humidifiers.* Although the oxygen output from indoor plants is not great, plants with large leaf surfaces that grow rapidly are capable of enhancing air quality. Attached greenhouses and atria filled with plants that effectively absorb carbon dioxide and oxygenate the air (spider plants do this very well) can improve the indoor environment while humidifying the air.

In the early 1990s, studies conducted at the John Stennis Space Center in Mississippi showed that plants can also act as effective filters. Former NASA scientist Bill C. Wolverton, Ph.D., has spent the past thirty years studying the ability of plants to clear volatile organic chemicals from indoor air. Wolverton predicts that within twenty years plants will be governmentally mandated in new buildings as a matter of public health.

According to the EPA, the most plentiful of the organic chemicals in the average indoor environment is formaldehyde. It is released from a host of household furnishings, including synthetic carpeting, particleboard (used to make bookcases, desks, and tables), foam insulation, upholstery, curtains, and even so-called air fresheners. Common houseplants such as chrysanthemums, striped dracaena, dwarf date palms, and especially Boston ferns are excellent filters for removing formaldehyde. Spider plants are also effective in removing carbon monoxide; areca palms are best at filtering xylene, the second most prevalent indoor organic chemical; and English ivy is good for filtering benzene, ranked third on the EPA's list. Aloe vera, philodendron, pothos, and ficus were also found to reduce levels of organic chemicals.

The Foliage for Clean Air Council, a communications clearinghouse for information on the use of foliage to improve indoor air quality, recommends a minimum of two plants per 100 square feet of floor space in an average home with eight- to ten-foot ceilings.

Prevention

Prevention of indoor air pollution involves eliminating pollutants at the source. Doctors who specialize in environmental medicine and some allergists can do skin and blood tests to help you identify pollutants to which you are particularly sensitive or allergic. These doctors are not always easy to find, nor are the tests always definitive, but they can help. With the use of environmentally sensitive architectural principles, a healthier home can be created. A major preventive strategy is the use of interior materials that emit no pollutants. Natural products such as wood, cotton, and metals are preferable to the lower-cost synthetic materials such as particleboard, fiberboard, polyester, and plastics.

Choosing to forgo a fireplace or wood-burning stove would be helpful, as would using a high-efficiency furnace with a sealed combustion unit to vent exhaust gases to the outside. Switch to nontoxic cleaning substances, including ordinary soap, vinegar, zephiran, and Air Therapy. (You can find a listing of such cleaners in *Nontoxic, Natural, and Earthwise,* by Debra Lynn Dadd.) Smoking should be relegated to the outdoors or to a well-ventilated enclosed space. If radon levels exceed the acceptable EPA standard of 4 picocuries per liter of air, radon control measures should be implemented. Formaldehyde from insulation can be eliminated by using the substitutes of cellulose and white fiberglass insulation.

BREATHING

Now that you've created optimum indoor air, let's look at how you might utilize it more efficiently. Oxygen is the most critical nutrient for every cell in the body. It is literally the "spark of life" needed to provide energy for every basic bodily function. Breathing is our constant and immediate connection to life: We can go days without water, weeks without food, but only minutes without oxygen. Headache is usually the first physical sign of a lack of oxygen. We begin life with our first breath and end it with our last. During our adult life we normally breathe about 23,000 times a day without ever giving much thought to this miraculous process.

Because respiration, synchronized with heartbeat, is an automatic function, we are seldom aware of how we breathe, or attempt to breathe more efficiently or healthfully, until we are confronted with the crisis of having great difficulty breathing, such as an asthma attack, being in a smoke-filled room, or at high altitude. These frightening, often terrifying, situations instantaneously alert us to the vital need for oxygen. Suddenly you become intimately aware of your own breath, your heart rate, muscle tension, your anxiety and fear. Your breath is labored, and you feel yourself fighting to breathe to save your life! The harder you struggle to breathe, the more rapid and shallow your breaths become, decreasing the available amount of oxygen. According to recent research, overbreathing—hyperventilation—might be a primary factor in triggering an asthmatic attack. It is well known that hyperventilation is also a common cause of headaches.

Whether cause or effect, most cases of backache are associated with shallow and more rapid breathing. Medical professor Konstantin Buteyko, a Russian researcher, has performed extensive experiments in Russia for over forty-five years on the effects of overbreathing. This led him to the controversial theory that hyperventilation is a primary *cause* of ailments such as asthma and headaches. He defines "hyperventilation" as the habitual inhalation of more than four to six liters of air per minute—considered to be the normal rate of respiration. It is the equivalent of eight to twelve breaths per minute, with each breath being the equivalent of a pint of air, or about two gallons per minute. In contrast, a person practiced in slow, rhythmic breathing may inhale five liters over a three-minute period, or a rate between three and four breaths per minute. With hyperventilation secondary to stress (a backache trigger), it can be as high as ten to fifteen liters during a one-minute period, as much as twenty to thirty breaths per minute. In addition to the lack of oxygen, this type of breathing also lowers carbon dioxide excessively.

Professor Buteyko recognized carbon dioxide not just as a waste product but as an important chemical regulator that is essential for the *utilization* of oxygen in the cells. Chronic overbreathing creates a deficiency of carbon dioxide, which decreases *available* oxygen, thus increasing the potential for muscle spasm (and back pain). By teaching patients techniques of slow, periodic under-breathing, he found that he could effect a significant reduction in asthma symptoms in 90 percent of his patients.

Teresa Hale, founder of the highly regarded Hale Clinic in London (the U.K.'s largest holistic medical clinic, with over one hundred practitioners, including thirty M.D.s), has confirmed Buteyko's findings and claims that his breathing techniques have produced dramatic reductions in asthma symptoms in just five days. She, too, found that it worked for 90 percent of their patients. She has proven similar success with applying the technique to headache sufferers. To my knowledge, no one has studied the effect of these breathing techniques on backache, but in my clinical practice I have found them to be quite helpful. To date, over 1 million people in the former Soviet Union have applied this technique with similar results on asthma. (For more in-depth information about Buteyko's method, refer to the book *Breathing Free* by Teresa Hale, listed in the Bibliography.)

These breathing techniques can be used for countering hyperventilation or in any situation where there is a lack of oxygen. Today, a growing number of researchers and practitioners are concluding that breathing techniques that emphasize the out breath, while breathing slowly and through the nose, are highly effective. Regardless of the cause, the lack of oxygen can provide you with an opportunity to learn how to intervene and consciously take control of breathing effectively. Obviously, learning to breathe more efficiently and taking in more oxygen are also important components in reducing backache and experiencing optimal health. You can choose to see your backache as being triggered by hyperventilation resulting from anxiety and stress, and as a warning your body is sending you. You can then use the experience as an opportunity to begin practicing more conscious and effective breathing—an act of loving your body. Breathing this way can help to break the cycle of anxiety and shortness of breath that accompany muscle tension and pain. As your lungs become better conditioned, practice becomes easier. Conscious breathing allows you to be much more in control and no longer a victim.

By learning to be more aware of your breathing patterns and applying a time-honored blend of traditional yogic techniques with newer, clinically proven methods, you will be able to lessen the frequency, duration, and intensity of backaches resulting from hyperventilation. Since stress is most often the trigger for hyperventilation, this type of breathing will help you to reduce stress and learn to relax.

In this chapter, I will coach you on a beginning level of breathing exercises. Consider this as the first step in putting your lungs into "breathing training camp" in order to condition them for consistently better function. You do not need to have back pain to benefit from these breathing techniques. The exercises help to strengthen peripheral and accessory breathing muscles that assist the lungs, thereby relieving the workload of the diaphragm. Most of us have an estimated 20 percent of unused lung capacity at any given time. When your lungs are trained to do so, you can draw on this reserve during times of respiratory distress.

Most people with backache have a heightened state of chronic muscle tension combined with exhaustion. This is because there is a long-term imbalance in the parasympathetic and sympathetic branches of the nervous system. The parasympathetic branch is like a "brake," creating relaxation, full and easy breathing, sleep, and good digestion. The sympathetic branch acts as the "accelerator." It rouses us to action and puts us into the "fight-or-flight" stress response when we perceive a threat. During the fight-or-flight response, adrenaline is released and breathing becomes shallow and rapid, heart rate and blood pressure go up, and muscles become tense in preparation for action. Many backache sufferers live highly stressed lives resulting in a condition of fight-or-flight breathing—a state of stressful, excessive sympathetic nervous function that can potentially exhaust the lungs and the adrenal glands. This state of sympathetic excess causes a form of chronic hyperventilation, or overbreathing, and leads to a constant state of *hypoxia,* low oxygen in the bloodstream. Hypoxia, in turn, can heighten anxiety and fatigue, which can significantly increase the frequency and intensity of backache.

Breathing Exercises

The Backache Survival approach to effective breathing techniques synthesizes the principles I have just discussed and starts you on three of the most important exercises. Remember to begin slowly, listen to your body's feedback, and practice at least once or twice a day for 5 minutes each time. (Many people choose to practice for a few minutes every hour. This is even more effective.) If for any reason you feel light-headed or out of breath, just take a minute or two to breathe normally and relax. Then try resuming the exercise again. If your sinuses are congested, then I recommend that you steam and do nasal irrigation prior to the exercises to open the nasal passages. If at all possible, try to perform these exercises in a clean air environment.

(1) *Basic Belly (or Abdominal) Breathing.* Begin by lying on your back with your knees up and legs slightly apart. Get comfortable and at first just notice your breathing without trying to do anything. Relax and feel yourself "sinking" into the floor. Then place your open hands around your lower rib cage with your palms at the lower part of your ribs and your fingertips touching at your belly button. Feel the

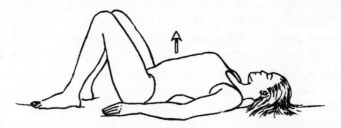

FIGURE 4.2

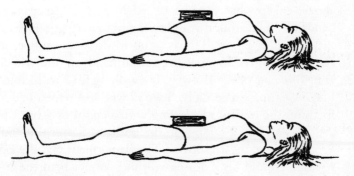

FIGURE 4.3

lower parts of your ribs expand and your belly rise up easily and smoothly as you breathe in through your nose. Now breathe out long and slow through your nose or mouth as you feel your belly sink. When breathing out through your mouth, keep your lips close together (but not completely closed), firmly pushing the air out. Try not to engage your shoulders or upper chest in the breathing effort. See if you can comfortably breathe out for 4 to 5 seconds or more, and in for 1 to 2 seconds. Go slowly, don't overbreathe, let the breath out long and slow while you relax and sink deeper into the floor. The out breath will relax you more and more. Breathing out will create air hunger and naturally encourage an inhalation. Let the in breath be slow, smooth, and through the nose. Feel the inhale deep in the back of your throat, *but do not take in a forced, large inhalation.* Remember that you want to emphasize a complete out breath. Try working toward breathing out for 8 to 12 seconds and in for 2 to 4. To feel your belly muscles even more, you may want to place a book or something that has some added weight on your abdomen for kinesthetic feedback. Once you are comfortable with this exercise add a variation: At the end of the out breath, try to hum, or add an *mmmm* or *nnnnn* sound to expel even more residual air.

(2) *Belly Breathing While Seated.* Use the same instructions as above, except that you are seated in a chair. Keep your hands wrapped around your lower ribs to get a good feel of the muscular action. This is good to do at the office, in class, even in traffic—but keep both hands on the wheel!

(3) *Belly Breathing While Walking.* Try walking for 5 to 15 minutes at a time, once daily. Start slowly and remember to focus on the out breath starting with a count of 4 out and 2 in. Try adding 2 counts on the out breath over time but keeping the in breath shorter. The basic rule is that the exhalation should be at least two times longer than the inhalation. Over a period of weeks or months, depending on your condition, try building the count on the out breath to

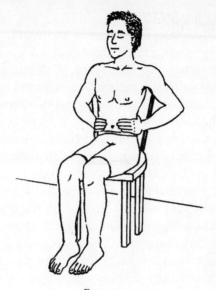

FIGURE 4.4

more than 10. Try adding a light hissing or whooshing sound from your lips while exhaling once you are tolerating the exercise well. Be patient and persistent. This helps condition the lungs for longer endurance and aerobic conditioning. Once you are tolerating this exercise well, you may want to try it on a mini-trampoline, also called a rebounder, while gently bouncing. The bouncing motion promotes lymphatic circulation and oxygenation.

Conditioned belly breathing can significantly help to reduce the intensity, duration, and frequency of your backaches. At the same time you will learn an effective method of relaxation while expanding your capacity to thrive, with much more energy and vitality and a greater sense of aliveness!

2. WATER AND MOISTURE

Next to oxygen, *water* is our most essential nutrient, and drinking enough water to satisfy your body's needs may be the simplest, least expensive (other than belly/abdominal breathing) self-help measure you can adopt to maintain your overall good health. Sufficient water can also help to prevent back pain by eliminating the often overlooked risk factor of dehydration. It has been estimated that 1 percent of dehydration in muscles can lead to an 8 to 10 percent energy loss in the muscles, thereby increasing the potential for spasm, pain, and tension.

Our adult bodies are 60 to 70 percent water (an infant's body is about 80 percent), and water is the medium through which every bodily function occurs. It is the basis of all body fluids, including blood, digestive juices, urine, lymph, and perspiration, which explains why we would die within a few days without water.

Water is vital to metabolism and digestion, and helps prevent both constipation and diarrhea. It is also critical to healthy nerve impulse conduction and brain function. Some of water's other vital functions in the body are:

- Enhancing oxygen uptake into the bloodstream (The surface of the lungs must be moistened with water to facilitate oxygen intake and the excretion of carbon dioxide.)
- Maintaining a high urine volume, helping to prevent kidney stones and urinary tract infections
- Regulating body temperature through perspiration
- Maintaining and increasing the health of the skin
- Maintaining adequate fluid for the lubrication of the joints and enhancing muscular function, particularly during and after exercise or other strenuous activity
- Moistening the mucous membranes of the respiratory tract, which in turn increases resistance to infection and thins the mucus, allowing it to drain more easily

WATER

Because water is so important to our health, all of us need to make a conscious effort to stay well hydrated, since most of us lose water faster than we replace it. For example, we lose one pint of water each day simply through exhalation. We also lose the same amount through perspiration, as well as three additional pints per day through urination and defecation. Exercise and heat exposure, especially in a dry climate, also increase water loss in the body. The percentage of body water content also decreases with age. All told, on average, each of us loses two and a half quarts of water (5 pints or 80 ounces) per day under normal conditions. Therefore, it is essential that the same amount or more be replenished daily.

Unfortunately, most Americans don't come close to consuming that much water per day. As a result, many of us are chronically dehydrated. When we think of dehydration, we may envision a lost soul in the desert, dying of thirst. However, most conditions of dehydration are not that dramatic, so that dehydration all too often is unsuspected and therefore undiagnosed. Meanwhile, its insidious effects can wreak havoc on our health by chronically impacting every one of our bodily functions, with the following results:

- Reduced blood volume, with less oxygen and nutrients provided to all muscles and organs
- Reduced brain size and impaired neuromuscular coordination, concentration, and thinking
- Excess body fat
- Poor muscle tone and size
- Impaired digestive function and constipation
- Increased toxicity in the body
- Joint and muscle pain
- Water retention (edema), which can result in a state of being overweight and also impede weight loss
- Hyperconcentration of blood with increased viscosity, leading to higher risk of heart attack

Even though you may not be feeling thirsty, you may none-theless be one of the millions of Americans who are chronically dehydrated. Observation of your urine is one simple way to determine if you are. If your urine is heavy, cloudy, and deep yellow, orange, or brown in tint, it's more than likely that you are dehydrated. The urine of a properly hydrated body tends to be light and nearly clear or whitish in color, similar in appearance to unsweetened lemonade. As your water intake approaches your daily need for it, you will notice the appearance of your urine changing accordingly. (Remember that B vitamins will also turn urine a dark yellow.)

Because dehydration is so deceptive—it can occur without symptoms of thirst—in general, we need to drink more water than our thirst calls for. This does not mean coffee, soft drinks, or alcohol, all of which further contribute to dehydration. Even processed fruit juices and milk are not healthy substitutes for water because of the sugar and possible pesticides in the former and the hormones and antibiotics in the latter.

The exact amount of water a person needs depends on a number of individual factors, such as body weight, diet, metabolic rate, climate, level of physical activity, and level of stress. Some health professionals recommend that we all drink eight 8-ounce glasses of water a day. A more accurate rule of thumb is to drink half an ounce of water per pound of body weight if you are a healthy but sedentary adult and to increase that amount to two thirds of an ounce per pound if you are an active exerciser. This means that a healthy, sedentary adult weighing 160 pounds should drink about ten 8-ounce glasses of water per day, while an active exerciser should drink thirteen to fourteen 8-ounce glasses. If your diet is particularly high in fresh fruits and vegetables, your daily water intake needs may be less, since these foods are 85 to 90 percent water in content and can help restore lost fluids. Herbal teas, natural fruit juices (without sugar added and diluted 50 percent with water), and soups that are sugarless and low in salt (the thinner the better) are also acceptable substitutes for drinking water.

Nearly as important as the amount of water you drink is the

quality of your water. Simply put, *if you aren't drinking filtered water, then your body is forced to become the filter.* Still, it's impossible to generalize about whether you should drink tap, bottled, or filtered water. (Distilled water is not recommended for drinking because it lacks necessary minerals and can also leach them from your body.) In some communities, water purity is so high that it requires no treatment, while other water sources are saturated with high concentrations of lead and radon, the two worst contaminants.

Another issue related to our drinking water is chlorination. Since chlorine was first introduced into America's drinking water supply in 1908, it has eliminated epidemics of cholera, dysentery, and typhoid. Multiple studies, however, now suggest an association between chlorine and increased free radical production, which can lead to a higher incidence of cancer. On the positive side, chlorine is effective in eliminating most microorganisms from drinking water. (One notable exception is the parasite *Cryptosporidium,* which is resistant to chlorine.)

Unless you live in one of the communities that supplies pure water, drinking tap water is not recommended, especially since the majority of health-related risks present in drinking water occur from contamination that is added *after* the water leaves the treatment and distribution plant. This includes pipes that run from municipal systems into your home, lead-soldered copper pipes, and fixtures that contain lead and may leach lead or other toxic metals (such as cadmium, mercury, and cobalt) into your tap water. Therefore, if you drink tap water, it would be a good idea to have the water from your tap tested, regardless of the claims from your local water utility. You can get started by calling your local health department for a referral for testing.

Because of the growing concerns regarding tap water, increasing numbers of Americans now choose bottled water for drinking and cooking purposes. This can not only prove to be expensive but also may not be as safe as you think. Regulations mandated for the bottled-water industry are similar to those followed by the public water treatment industry and currently do not include required testing for *Cryptosporidium* and many other contaminants. Moreover, 25 percent of bottled water sold in this country comes from filtered municipal water that is then treated. For this reason, perhaps the healthiest choice regarding your drinking water is to invest in a water filter. Reverse-osmosis filters appear to be the most effective home water-filtering systems presently available. But there are also some distillation and carbon filters that are able to reduce lead in water significantly. There are carafe-style filters for the kitchen faucet that cost about $25, under-the-sink models for $400, and point-of-entry units that purify the water as it enters the house. These can cost as much as $1,250.

Since it is impossible to know with certainty whether what you drink or eat is completely safe, do the best you can. To get in the habit of drinking enough water, spread your intake throughout the day (drinking very little after dinner), and don't drink more than four 8-ounce glasses in any one-hour period. It's also best to drink between meals so as not to interfere with your body's digestive process. Make your water drinking convenient; keep a container of water at hand, in your car, or at your desk, and don't wait until you feel thirsty to start drinking. Most important, be sure that there's always a bathroom nearby. The belief that you can stretch your bladder is a myth.

HUMIDIFICATION

According to Dr. Marshall Plaut, chief of the asthma and allergy branch at the National Institute of Allergy and Infectious Diseases (part of the National Institutes of Health), "Dry air triggers asthma and nasal congestion." I, too, have been convinced for quite some time that dry air, and especially cold and dry air, is a major contributor to asthma, sinusitis, and bronchitis. As a chronic irritant to the sensitive nasal mucous membranes, dry air can also contribute to a greater susceptibility to allergies. Studies on patients with allergic rhinitis have shown that warm, moist air can improve nasal congestion and other allergy symptoms.

Optimum indoor air quality requires air containing between

35 and 55 percent relative humidity. Moisture provided by room humidifiers can greatly benefit anyone with a respiratory condition. These humidifiers are most helpful in the winter, even in humid, cold-weather climates, because most heating systems dry the indoor air considerably. However, if you are sensitive to mold, then I would be more cautious about using a humidifier.

If you rarely suffer jolts of static electricity when you touch metal objects such as doorknobs, then the air in your home is probably humid enough. For a more precise test, you'll need a hygrometer. You can find these humidity measuring devices at most hardware stores. The one I've been using is the Bionaire Climate Check, a digital device that measures both temperature and humidity.

Room humidifiers, also called tabletop models, have sufficient capacity to humidify a medium- to large-size room. Each type has some drawbacks. Ultrasonic models can emit an irritating white dust. So can cool-mist models, which require the use of distilled water or an expensive demineralization cartridge, unless you have very soft water. Steam-mist models, also called vaporizers, can scald if you get too close to the mist they produce or if you tip them over by accident. Evaporative models, the most prevalent type, can become a breeding ground for bacteria. Warm-mist units are my first choice. They produce a mist just slightly warmer than room air, use tap water, require no filter, and are able to kill bacteria. Their only drawback may be that they use more electricity than the other types. Most humidifiers are quiet and very effective in producing a moist environment in an enclosed space. They are available in pharmacies, department stores, and hardware stores under a variety of brand names. The one I know best and with which I have enjoyed excellent results is the Bionaire-Clear Mist 5 (CMP-5). It quietly yet powerfully puts out warm moisture, can cover an area of up to 1,600 square feet, and is relatively easy to clean. The Kenmore Warm Mist is the identical unit, and it is available at most Sears stores. These units cost about $125. Although the ideal humidifier has probably not yet been designed, I've recently tried and am pleased with the Slant/Fin GF-200. This warm-mist humidifier uses ultraviolet germicidal technology to produce 99.999 percent germ-free mist. It costs under $100. The room or tabletop humidifiers can cost from $30 to $125.

The larger humidifiers, called consoles, can humidify an average-size house, cost from $100 to $200, and are all the evaporative type. Although I've had no personal experience with these, I know that *Consumer Reports* has given a high rating to the Bionaire W-6S, as well as to the Toastmaster 3435 and the Emerson HD850.

Central or in-duct humidifiers, those that attach to the furnace, are more convenient but often do not humidify an individual room as well as a portable humidifier can when the door to the room is closed. In the past, the major problem with central humidifiers was that most of them were the reservoir type, with a tray of standing water that breeds mold and bacteria. I recommend the flow-through type of central humidifier, such as Aprilaire or General, which eliminates the stagnant-water problem and is easy to maintain. Depending on the model, size of your home, and installation, this humidifier would probably cost about $250 to $650.

Humidifiers are not the only option for moisturizing your home. The installation of waterfalls, indoor spas, and swimming pools will all add a lot of moisture to the house, but, of course, they are expensive to install and maintain. It may surprise you to learn that even the moisture from human breath and sweat, along with that from cooking, baths, showers, and plants, adds significantly to a home's humidity. If your bedroom is dry, hang a wet towel on a hanger in the room.

Another device I've been using preventively on myself and recommending to patients is the *steam inhaler.* It can be quite soothing to dry and irritated mucous membranes while also relieving sinus headaches. There is evidence that steam also helps to open your airways and can act as a decongestant and bronchodilator. A few drops or a spray of medicinal eucalyptus oil added to the unit while you are steaming enhances its therapeutic effect. For quick relief of a sinus headache, I often recommend spraying this eucalyptus (Sinus Survival Eucalyptus Spray) on a tissue held close to the nose while inhaling through the nose. To benefit the entire mucous membrane while steaming, alternate inhaling through your nose (upper respiratory tract) and your mouth (lower respiratory tract—lungs). If used just prior to nasal irrigation, it will greatly increase the benefit of the irrigation. The steam inhaler I use is made by Kaz and costs about $50, but unfortunately is no longer readily available. Complete information on where to obtain any of the products I mention is listed in the Product Index at the end of the book. For additional information on treating chronic sinusitis, please refer to the fourth edition of *Sinus Survival*.

Assuming your environment is relatively dry, as indoor air tends to be during the winter months in most parts of the United States, you can also provide moisture with a *saltwater* (also called *saline*) *nasal spray*. There are several commercial products available in pharmacies. However, you can make your own saline spray by mixing ½ teaspoon of noniodized table salt and a pinch of baking soda in an 8-ounce cup of lukewarm bottled water (without chlorine) and dispensing it from a spray bottle. I'd suggest using sea salt without iodine. Spray into each nostril while closing off the other nostril and simultaneously inhaling. This is nonaddictive and can be done as often as you like throughout the day. It has no negative side effects, except for the curious looks you will get from those wanting to know what you are spraying in your nose.

The Sinus Survival Nasal Spray, a botanical saline nasal mist, has been a highly effective addition to the Sinus Survival Program. Formulated by Dr. Steve Morris, a naturopathic physician from Mukilteo, Washington, and myself, we have been using it ourselves and recommending it to our patients for almost ten years, with excellent results. In addition to saline, which makes up the bulk of the spray, the ingredients include three medicinal herbs that are soothing and healing to the nasal mucous membranes.

- *Goldenseal*—acts as an antibacterial, antifungal, and anti-inflammatory

- *Aloe vera*—has antifungal properties and relieves irritation
- *Grapefruit-seed extract*—an excellent antifungal

The Sinus Survival Nasal Spray is available in many health food stores and can also be obtained through Sinus Survival Services.

An even more effective way of moisturizing is *saline irrigation*. This procedure can result in dramatic relief from pain by reducing swelling in the nasal passages, causing a reduction of pressure in the sinus, as well as helping to empty the sinus of its infected mucus. Saltwater sprays also irrigate—that is, wash out—some mucus, bacteria, and dust particles, while reducing swelling. However, they don't do it as well as the following irrigation methods. Throughout the past decade I've heard many people comment that nasal irrigation, using any of the first three techniques described below, has been the *single most helpful component* of the entire Sinus Survival Program. Irrigation should be done three to four times a day for acute sinusitis and once or twice for a milder chronic condition. Many former sinus sufferers continue to irrigate daily on a preventive basis, even after curing their chronic sinusitis.

Mix the saline solution for irrigation fresh each day in 1 cup of lukewarm bottled water. Add ½ teaspoon of noniodized table salt or sea salt and a tiny pinch of baking soda, thus making the solution close to normal body fluid salinity and pH. (Irrigating with plain water is usually somewhat uncomfortable.) Use the full cup of saline solution for each irrigation (one-half cup for each nostril). Lean over the sink, with the head rotated so that the nostril to be irrigated is directly above the other nostril, while using one of the following methods. Always blow your nose *very gently* after irrigating.

Method 1   For the past eight years, I have been recommending the use of the Neti Pot and, more recently, SinuCleanse, for nasal irrigation. It is a small porcelain pot with a narrow spout (SinuCleanse is plastic with a very similar shape and size). This is probably the most gentle and convenient method for irrigation.

Because of this, people with chronic sinusitis are much more apt to use this method on a regular basis, both therapeutically in treating an infection and preventively. SinuCleanse is sold with packets of hypertonic saline to mix with water, making this method even more convenient. The Neti Pot is made by the Himalayan Institute in Honesdale, Pennsylvania, and is available in many health food stores. SinuCleanse is available through Thriving Health Products.

Method 2   Use an angled nasal irrigator attachment (the Grossan Nasal Irrigator is available at some pharmacies) on a Waterpik® appliance. Set the Waterpik at the *lowest* possible pressure and insert the irrigator tip just inside one nostril, pinching your nostril to form a seal. Irrigate with your mouth open, allowing the fluid to drain out of your mouth or nose. Repeat the procedure in the other nostril. The pulsations of the Waterpik make this perhaps the most effective method for irrigation. However, it is also the most expensive. In November 2002, Dr. Grossan introduced a new irrigation device called the Hydro-Pulse® Nasal Irrigator. Similar to the Waterpik, it has been designed specifically for nasal irrigation and is currently the most effective method I'm aware of.

Method 3   Completely fill a large, all-rubber ear syringe (available at most pharmacies) with saline solution. Lean over the sink and insert the syringe tip just inside one nostril, so that it forms a comfortable seal. *Gently* squeeze and release the bulb several times to swish the solution around the inside of your nose. The solution will run out both nostrils and may also run out of your mouth. Repeat this for each nostril until one cup of saline solution is used or until the solution is clear.

Method 4   For very small children, irrigate with 10 to 20 drops of saline solution per nostril from an eyedropper.

If you are using a decongestant nasal spray or a corticosteroid nasal spray, use them only *after* the saltwater nasal irrigations.

These methods obviously require more effort than the saline nasal sprays, but many patients comment on how much more helpful they are.

Another solution that has been effective in irrigation is called Alkalol. It is a mucus solvent and cleaner and can be used with the saline solution in a 1:1 ratio (one-half saline, one-half Alkalol) with all of the methods previously mentioned. You will probably have to ask your pharmacist to order it for you, as it is usually not in stock, but Alkalol is very inexpensive.

Although I realize that the vast majority of the readers of this book are suffering from chronic back pain, I strongly believe that a healthy respiratory tract is needed to obtain a maximal supply of oxygen. This in turn will significantly benefit your back. That's why I think it's important to have included as much detailed information about moisture, humidification, and maintaining healthy mucous membranes as I have. You may not choose to follow any of these suggestions, but if you're congested and not breathing freely, then I'd strongly recommended trying at least some of them.

3. FOOD AND SUPPLEMENTS

DIET

There is not one universal diet that ideally suits every individual. Certain functional lab tests, a comprehensive nutritional history, and personal experimentation (trial and error), along with the guidance of a holistic physician, can assist you in determining the diet best suited to your unique requirements. The following guidelines, however, are self-care approaches to establishing a diet for which almost anyone can derive significant health benefits.

The relationship of a healthy diet to health has been emphasized for centuries in both the East and West. While proper diet alone may not be enough to entirely reverse certain types of disease (this is true of backache), most chronic medical conditions can be significantly improved by a diet of nutrient-rich foods and adequate intake of purified water. Unfortunately, our society, with its overreliance on fast foods and snacks, affords great temptation to stray from healthy eating habits. And even when we do resolve to change our diet for the better, many of us wind up confused about what foods to actually eat and how they should be prepared, due in great part to the steady introduction of best-selling books touting the "latest and greatest" cure-all diet. While such books may be well intentioned, not all of them contain scientifically supported recommendations, and those that do often contradict equally researched and published information that made the best-seller's list the year before. As a result, a number of polls now indicate that growing numbers of Americans are literally "fed up" with the amount of dietary and nutritional information that is becoming increasingly available in our society.

A good dose of common sense can go a long way toward alleviating this confusion. There is a great deal of truth to the old adage, "You are what you eat." The foods you consume become the fuel your body uses to carry out its countless functions. Therefore, it makes good sense to eat those foods that are the best "fuel sources." This means foods that are rich in vitamins, minerals, enzymes, essential fatty and amino acids, and other necessary nutrients, free of preservatives, pesticides, and other substances that deplete the body's energy and can damage vital organs. Dr. Todd Nelson's (a Denver naturopathic doctor and co-author of several of my books) recommended diet, the *New Life Eating Plan* (NLEP), is the one I follow and suggest to my patients.

Phase I of the NLEP, described below, beginning on page 106, outlines the initial stages of rebalancing body chemistry to help restore optimal function and heal your backache. Phase I serves as the basis of healthy eating for those who are experiencing chronic illness. Phase II, at the end of this section (page 126), allows for some dietary expansion and food rotation.

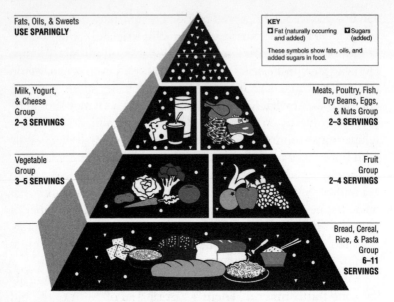

Food Guide Pyramid

Rethinking the American Way of Eating

In January 1992, the U.S. Department of Agriculture (USDA) unveiled its recommended dietary pyramid as a guideline for meeting these nutritional needs. At the base of this pyramid are whole grains, such as brown rice, bulgur, wheat (breads and pasta), oats, barley, millet, and cereals, with a recommended 6 to 11 servings from this food group per day. The next section of the pyramid is divided into the categories of fruits (with a recommended 2 to 4 servings) and vegetables (with a recommended 3 to 5 servings). Moving upward, we find a recommended 2 to 3 servings each of dairy products (milk, yogurt, and cheese), and the meats, poultry, fish, dry beans, eggs, and nuts group; with fats, oils, and sweets at the top to be used sparingly.

While the USDA food pyramid can be a useful place to start, a number of recent studies now indicate that our daily need for carbohydrates from whole grains may not be as vital as our need for fresh fruits and vegetables. A good deal of this research has been popularized by Dr. Barry Sears, Ph.D., in his diet book, *The Zone*. He and other researchers have found that there are a variety of harmful effects resulting from excessive intake of carbohydrates, especially those that have a high *glycemic index* (they break down quickly and release glucose into the blood at a rapid rate). These ill effects include:

- Overstimulation of insulin production, which can lead to excess storage of fat in the body, hypoglycemia, increased inflammation, cardiac risk, and diabetes
- Diminished physical and mental capacity
- Fluctuating energy levels and mood swings
- Predisposition to chronic diseases, including arthritis, heart disease, and skin disorders

As a result, practitioners of holistic medicine now place more emphasis on the fruit and vegetable groups, recommending more servings of these two food groups over whole grains, breads, pasta, and cereal. Flour-based food—bread, pasta, and bagels—have a very high glycemic index. Whole grains, beans and legumes, and most starchy vegetables, except potatoes, have a low glycemic index and are emphasized in the NLEP. (See Table 4.2, the Glycemic Index, on pages 92–94.)

It is also recommended that milk—other than 1 percent fat or skim—and margarine be eliminated and that your daily intake of butter and cheese be reduced.

Beyond the USDA Food Pyramid

Dr. Nelson developed the NLEP after realizing that all of his chronically ill patients were making at least six critical dietary mistakes. These six were part of a list that he identified as the fifteen most common mistakes in the American diet that undermine health. They are:

(1) Excess saturated fat, trans-fats, cooked fats, and insufficient essential fatty acids (EFAs)

Table 4.2

Glycemic Index

Carbohydrates act like a powerful drug elevating insulin in the body. This in turn can increase fat deposits, LDL cholesterol (the unhealthy kind), and inflammation, while decreasing immunity. The amount of insulin the body produces is based on the amount of carbohydrates that actually enters the bloodstream as the simple sugar glucose. This is why you can consume a large amount of the 3 percent or 6 percent vegetables and fruits (refer to Table 4.3, Carbohydrate Classifications of Fruits and Vegetables, page 94) in comparison to the amount of grains, starches, breads, or pastas at any given meal.

Example: 1½ cups of broccoli, or any other 3-percent vegetable = ¼ cup pasta.

This is why it is best to focus on the low-density carbohydrates (3 percent and 6 percent). Not only can you eat more, but there are many other benefits, including high water content, high fiber content, vitamins, minerals, and enzymes.

People are genetically designed to eat primarily fruits and vegetables as their major source of carbohydrates.

All carbohydrates, simple or complex, have to be broken down into simple sugars before being absorbed by the body and entering the bloodstream. The only simple sugar that can actually enter the bloodstream is glucose. The faster glucose enters the bloodstream, the more insulin you make. This is important for you to know when you are making your choice of carbohydrates. *The higher the glycemic index of carbohydrates, the faster it enters the bloodstream as sugar.*

Low Glycemic (Examples: 3-percent and 6-percent fruits and vegetables)

Fructose has to be converted into glucose via the liver, so fruits are a lower glycemic index than grains and starches.

High Glycemic (Examples: bagel, pasta, cooked starches)

Cornflakes are pure glucose linked by chemical bonds. These bonds are easily broken in the stomach, and glucose rushes into the bloodstream. Table sugar is one-half glucose and one-half fructose, so it actually enters the bloodstream slower than a bagel.

There are other factors involved that have an effect on how fast the carbohydrates are broken down into simple sugar. Fat and soluble fibers slow the entry of glucose. Soluble fiber is an important distinction. There are two types of fiber, soluble (pectin, apples) and insoluble (cellulose, bran cereal). And because fat slows down the entry of glucose into the bloodstream, the sugar in ice cream actually is absorbed more slowly than that of a bagel. High fiber in low glycemic foods is the slowest to release sugars.

The more the carbohydrates are cooked, the higher the glycemic index will be. This is because the cell structure is broken down by cooking and processing. The glycemic index is dramatically increased in instant foods made from rice and potatoes. Therefore all bread has a high glycemic index.

Highest Glycemic Index Foods
(Examples: puffed cereal and puffed rice cakes)
The body needs a constant intake of carbohydrates for optimal brain function. Too much carbohydrate and the body increases insulin secretion to drive down blood sugar. Too little and the brain will not function efficiently. (High glycemic food should always be avoided with candida overgrowth.)

Remember, protein stimulates glucagon, which reduces insulin secretion, while fat and fiber slow down the rate of entry of any carbohydrate.

(2) Excess sweets
(3) Excess refined carbohydrates and insufficient complex carbohydrates
(4) Excess alcohol
(5) Excess caffeine
(6) Excess salt
(7) Excess consumption of overly cooked food
(8) Excess processed and devitalized food
(9) Excess "high stress" protein sources and insufficient "low stress" protein sources
(10) Excess consumption of food-born toxins (preservatives, additives, artificial sweeteners, colorings, flavorings, hydrogenated fats)

Table 4.3

Carbohydrate Classifications of Fruits and Vegetables (According to Carbohydrate Content)

VEGETABLES

3%	6%	15%	20+%
asparagus	beans, string	artichoke	beans, dried
bean sprouts	beets	carrot	beans, lima
beet greens	brussels sprouts	oyster plant	corn
broccoli	chives	parsnip	potato, sweet
cabbage	collard greens	peas, green	potato, white
cauliflower	dandelion greens	squash	yam
celery	eggplant		
chard, swiss	kale		
cucumber	kohlrabi		
endive	leek		
lettuce	okra		
mustard greens	onion		
radish	parsley		
spinach	pepper, red		
watercress	pimento		
	pumpkin		
	rutabagas		
	turnip		

FRUITS

3%	6%	15%	20+%
cantaloupe	apricot (fresh only)	apple	banana
melons	blackberries	grapes	figs
rhubarb	blueberries	kumquats	prunes
strawberries	cherries	loganberries	or any dried
tomato	cranberries	mango	fruit
	grapefruit	mulberries	watermelon
	guava	pear	
	kiwi	pineapple (fresh)	
	lemon	pomegranate	
	lime		
	melons		
	orange		
	papaya		
	peach		
	plum		
	raspberries		
	tangerine		

(11) Insufficient high-quality, fresh organic produce—both fruits and vegetables
(12) Insufficient pure water
(13) Insufficient balanced fiber intake
(14) Poor food combinations
(15) Stressful eating environment and insufficient chewing

Consistently making poor choices in these fifteen areas over the course of a lifetime will usually result in poor health. This occurs from the cumulative effect of increased chemical toxicity, free radical damage, nutrient depletion, and dysbiosis, resulting in immune, endocrine, neurologic, rheumatologic, and cardiac dysfunction.

Dr. Nelson has concluded that the goal of any dietary program for preventing and treating a chronic illness should be correcting these common mistakes and establishing a regenerative way of eating for life. This is the primary purpose of the New Life Eating Plan. As you begin to adopt these principles, you'll soon realize that this diet is an essential component of the daily practice of loving and nurturing yourself.

Let's now explore some of the specific steps you can take in committing to the NLEP. Out of the fifteen most common mistakes, we will emphasize changing the first six from the list above. These are perhaps the most important mistakes that we commonly make, which we refer to as "the sickening six."

THE SICKENING SIX

There are six substances in the American diet that should be substantially eliminated—unhealthy fats, sugar, refined carbohydrates, alcohol, caffeine, and salt. These "sickening six" can lead to a variety of disease conditions. While it is acceptable to enjoy these substances in moderation, keeping their intake to a minimum can pay big health dividends. Here are a number of reasons why.

1. Unhealthy Fats

The regular intake of good fats is essential to our health. Unfortunately, most of us are getting too much unhealthy fat in our diets. Primary sources of these harmful fats include red meats, milk and other dairy products, and the hydrogenated trans-fats found in margarine, cooking fats, and many brands of peanut butter. These fats are also found in many packaged foods, including most commercial cereals, which also tend to be loaded with sugar.

A regular intake of excess "bad" fat directly contributes to inflammation of any kind and therefore can contribute to, and prolong, back pain. Bad fats act as triggers for an avalanche of inflammatory chemicals that can cause muscle soreness, spasms, and joint pain.

Unhealthy fats lead to arteriosclerosis and the buildup of plaque on the inner lining of the arteries, which over time can obstruct the flow of blood and the transport of oxygen and nutrients to the body's internal organs. This obstruction, in turn, can lead to heart attacks, angina, stroke, kidney failure, and pregangrene in the legs. The excessive intake of unhealthy fats is also associated with certain cancers. Among them are cancer of the breast, colon, rectum, prostate, ovaries, and uterus. This is particularly true of the saturated fats derived from meat products.

Obesity, which is increasing to epidemic proportions in this country, is also directly related to excessive fat (and sugar) intake. Obesity is a primary cause of low back pain because being overweight puts undue stress on both the low back and abdominal muscles. Obesity is a serious disease condition by itself, but, if prolonged, it can contribute to many other forms of illness, including adult-onset diabetes.

Becoming aware of your fat intake and minimizing the amount of harmful fats you consume are important steps toward optimal health.

2. Sugar

The use of sugar in your diet can pose many harmful health risks, yet the average American consumes 150 pounds each year. This is the equivalent of over 40 teaspoons of sugar every day. The following are only a few of sugar's health-depleting effects.

- Sugar has been shown to be a risk factor for heart disease *and may be more harmful than fat.*
- Sugar weakens the immune system, increasing susceptibility to infection and allergy and further exacerbating all other diseases caused by diminished immune function.
- Sugar stimulates excessive insulin production, thereby causing more fat to be stored in the body; lowers HDL cholesterol levels (the healthy cholesterol); increases the production of harmful triglycerides; and increases the risk of arteriosclerosis (hardening of the arteries). When insulin is regularly secreted in high levels, it becomes pro-inflammatory: it fans the flames on any type of inflammation, including back pain.
- Sugar contributes to diminished mental capacity and can cause feelings of anxiety, depression, and rage. It has also been implicated in certain cases of attention deficit disorder (ADD).
- High sugar intake is associated with certain cancers, including cancer of the gall bladder and colon. Recently, sugar has also been implicated as a causative factor in cases of breast cancer.
- Excessive sugar in the diet is a primary contributor to candidiasis (intestinal yeast overgrowth), which can lead to a host of health problems, including gastrointestinal disorders, asthma, bronchitis, sinusitis, allergies, and chronic fatigue.

If you still feel a need to satisfy your sweet tooth, substitute modest amounts of pure honey, maple syrup, or the herb stevia to decrease the risk of these adverse effects.

3. Refined Carbohydrates

Refined, or simple, carbohydrates, such as those found in white breads and pastas made from white flour, are another group of health-threatening agents. When eaten to excess, these types of foods overstimulate insulin production and produce the same excessive fat storage in the body that results from eating too much sugar. This can lead to the onset of diabetes and obesity. The rise in obesity among American children is due in part to a diet heavy in sugars and refined carbohydrates and deficient in nutritious alternatives, notably fruits and vegetables.

Several recent studies have shown that certain carbohydrates previously promoted as being "whole" sources of starch are very rapidly digested and absorbed. As a result, they elevate blood sugar fully as much as sugar itself, contributing to all of the problems cited above (see Sugar). Most carbohydrates have been carefully analyzed and assigned a *glycemic index* rating (for a rating of fruits and vegetables, refer to page 94). A high glycemic index indicates that a food acts much like sugar in the body, while food sources with a low glycemic index are much slower to be assimilated and therefore offer much better nutritional value. High glycemic index foods include cornflakes, puffed rice, rice cakes, instant and mashed potatoes, white bread, maltose, and, of course, sugar itself. Foods with a low glycemic index include whole grain cereals (oats, brown rice, amaranth, quinoa, kamut, millet), legumes (beans, peas, peanuts, soybeans), pumpernickel breads, rye crackers, whole wheat pastas, pearled barley, bulgur wheat, brown rice, sweet potatoes, apples, and unsweetened/plain yogurt.

4. Alcohol

Alcohol is another example of a substance that, when taken in moderation, may enhance health, but when consumed in excess can cause a variety of serious problems. A growing body of research now indicates that one or two beers or a glass of wine per day can be beneficial to health as a way to relieve stress and to improve digestion. In fact, studies have shown that complete ab-stainers from alcohol have a slightly shorter life expectancy than those who drink moderate amounts. Unfortunately, for many men especially, alcohol and moderation usually "don't mix."

Although most people drink in order to feel better, evidence indicates that excessive alcohol can significantly contribute to feelings of depression, loneliness, restlessness, and boredom, ac-cording to studies conducted by the National Center for Health Statistics. In addition, very moody people are also three times as likely to be heavy drinkers (three or more drinks per day).

Aside from the social stigma surrounding excessive alcohol consumption, too much alcohol can also contribute to obesity; increased blood pressure; diabetes; colon, stomach, breast, mouth, esophageal, laryngeal, and pancreatic cancers; gastrointestinal disorders; impaired liver function; candidiasis; impaired mental functioning; and behavioral and emotional dysfunctions. If you are having difficulty in bringing your alcohol consumption under control, seek the help of a professional counselor.

5. Caffeine

Caffeine is a drug to which more than half of all Americans are addicted. On average, we drink at least 2½ cups of coffee a day, or 425 mg of caffeine. Because caffeine acts as a stimulant, we con-sume it in order to have more energy. But the quick-fix boost it provides usually only lasts for a few hours, leaving us with greater fatigue and irritability once its effects wear off. Typically, when this happens, we reach for another cup of coffee to keep us going. The result is a roller coaster of ups and downs, which, over time, can result in a number of health hazards.

While caffeine in moderation (200 mg or less per day) is rel-atively safe, the regular consumption of greater amounts can re-sult in elevated blood pressure; increased risk of cancer, heart disease, and osteoporosis; poor sleep patterns; anxiety and irri-tability; dizziness; impaired circulation; urinary frequency; and gastrointestinal disorders. Caffeine also causes muscle cells to lose calcium and can interfere with the blood clotting process by decreasing platelet stickiness.

Taken in moderation, however, caffeine has been shown to enhance mental functioning and to improve both alertness and mood, suggesting that 200 mg or less of caffeine per day may be safely tolerated by most individuals.

If you consider yourself addicted to caffeine, the best way to break your habit is to reduce your intake *very gradually,* over a period of a few weeks or even months. Start by substituting non-caffeinated drinks such as herbal tea or a roasted grain beverage in place of one of your normal cups of coffee per day. Over time, cut back further while increasing the number of substitute beverages, and beware of possible withdrawal symptoms such as headache, nervousness, and irritability. Typically, these will pass within a day or two. Also avoid other caffeine sources, such as soft drinks (particularly colas), cocoa, chocolate, and nonherbal teas. If you still choose to drink coffee, the least harmful choice is Swiss water–processed organic decaffeinated coffee.

CAFFEINE AMOUNTS (MG)

Coffee (5-ounce cup)

Decaffeinated instant: 2
Decaffeinated brewed: 2–5
Instant: 65–100
Percolated: 65–125
Drip: 115–175

Tea (5-ounce cup)

Bag, brewed for five minutes: 20–60
Bag, brewed for one minute: 10–40
Loose, black, five-minute brew: 20–85
Loose, green, five-minute brew: 15–80
Iced: 25–70

Soft drinks (12-ounce glass)

Cola: 45
Mountain Dew: 55

Chocolate

Cocoa, 5-ounce cup: 4–6
Milk chocolate, 1 ounce: 3–6
Bittersweet chocolate, 1 ounce: 25–35

6. Salt

Salt is another ingredient that is far too prevalent in many diets, and it poses particular dangers for certain people who suffer from high blood pressure. Many of us have been conditioned since childhood to crave salt, but its overuse draws water into the bloodstream. This, in turn, increases blood volume, causing higher blood pressure levels. Too much salt also upsets the body's sodium-potassium balance, thereby interfering with the lymphatic system's ability to draw wastes away from the cells.

Although some salt can be used in cooking, a good rule of thumb is to avoid adding salt to your food once it is served.

BEGINNING THE NLEP

As a starting point in changing your diet, reduce your intake of red meat, and when you do eat it, choose only the leanest cuts. In its place, have two to three servings per day of either fish, poultry, beans, or nuts. Also avoid all cooking fats and oils derived from animal products and those from vegetable sources that are hydrogenated and found in most margarines, many brands of peanut butter, and hydrogenated cooking fats. Instead, use vegetable oils such as olive or canola. Flaxseed oil, a particularly rich source of vital omega-3 essential fatty acids, can also be used in dressings (but not for cooking). The best fats are unprocessed, polyunsaturated, and non-oxidized, and are derived from whole nuts and seeds, fish, vegetables, and grains.

Also pay attention to the various food additives that are commonly found in the typical American diet. These include all chemical preservatives, such as BHA, BHT, sodium nitrate, and sulfites; artificial coloring agents; and artificial sweeteners such as saccharin, aspartame (Nutrasweet), and cyclamates. These additives have the potential to be enormous health risks. To avoid their use, stay away from processed or canned foods and get in the habit of reading labels whenever you go shopping. As a rule, if you can't pronounce the ingredient, don't eat it.

Finally, if you aren't already accustomed to doing so, consider selecting fruits and vegetables that are grown organically and meats and poultry derived from animals that are raised free-range. In the former case, you will be eating foods that are richer in nutrients and free of pesticides, artificial fertilizers, preservatives, and other additives. Free-range meats and poultry are the end products of animals that are not subject to injections of growth hormones, antibiotics, and irradiation commonly found in meats and poultry raised commercially.

What follows, by category, are listings of a variety of nutritious foods that can be added to your diet for their rich nutrient value.

Fruits and Vegetables

Fresh fruits and vegetables, organic when possible, should be a staple of your daily diet. Not only are they rich with nutrients but also possess vital cleansing properties and high fiber content, which help rid the body of waste and toxins, creating greater levels of energy. Be sure to eat at least part of your daily servings of fruits and vegetables raw, since in this form you will be receiving the highest nutrient content. Lightly steaming vegetables is another healthy way to prepare them. Boiling or overcooking vegetables can destroy the abundant vitamins, minerals, and enzymes in these foods. Have a goal of eating three to six cups of vegetables daily, mostly at lunch and dinner. In addition, eat two to three servings of fruit between meals as snacks.

Among the fruits and vegetables with the greatest nutritional value (especially vitamin C and carotenes) are blueberries, cherries, red grapes, plums, oranges, cantaloupe, strawberries, apples, guavas, red chili peppers, red and green sweet peppers, kale, parsley, greens (mustard, collard, and turnip), broccoli, cauliflower, brussels sprouts, carrots, yams, spinach, mangoes, winter squash, romaine lettuce, asparagus, tomatoes, onions, garlic, mushrooms, peaches, papayas, bananas, watermelon, and sprouts.

Note: Although they are extremely rich sources of vitamins, minerals, and fiber, fruits impede the digestion of other foods and are therefore best eaten away from meals as snacks: 10 or more minutes before or 2 hours after a meal.

Whole Grains and Complex Carbohydrates

Whenever possible, whole grains, beans, and legumes should be your primary source of carbohydrates as they, too, provide many essential vitamins and minerals. Most grains also supply about 10 percent of excellent quality protein. Among the recommended whole grains are amaranth, millet, brown rice, basmati rice, quinoa, barley, rye, and oats. Use wheat sparingly, on a rotation basis, according to NLEP Phase II (see page 126). Other sources of complex carbodyrates are starchy vegetables and legumes. Complex carbohydrates provide sustained boosts of energy and digest slowly, releasing their sugars into the bloodstream gradually. This gradual release of sugars helps to maintain insulin balance and contributes to the production of *adenosine triphosphate* (ATP) in the cells, thereby strengthening the immune system. Good sources of starchy vegetables include sweet potatoes, yams, acorn and butternut squash, and pumpkins. For legumes, choose black beans, garbanzo beans (chick peas), lima beans, adzuki beans, navy beans, kidney beans, lentils, black-eyed peas, and split peas.

Proteins

Proteins are the nutrients your body uses to build cells, repair tissue, and produce the basic building blocks of DNA and RNA. Bones, hair, nails, muscle fibers, collagen, and other connective tissues are all composed of protein, and protein itself is second only to water in terms of the body's overall composition.

The main sources of protein for a healthy diet are ocean fish, chicken and turkey (select cuts that are free-range and free of hormones and antibiotics), healthy eggs, soy products (soy milk, tofu, miso, and tempeh), sunflower seeds, almonds, cashews, pine nuts, pecans, walnuts, and sesame seeds. Red meats and dairy products are not on this list due to their higher concentration of unhealthy fats, which can contribute to a host of disease conditions, especially heart disease and hardening of the arteries. Low- or nonfat cultured dairy products such as yogurt or cottage cheese are well tolerated by many people.

Fats and Oils

Contrary to popular belief, all of us need a certain amount of fat in our diet. Fats supply energy reserves that the body draws upon when not enough fat is present in the foods we eat. Fats also serve as a primary form of insulation and help to maintain normal body temperature. In addition, fats help to transport oxygen; absorb fat-soluble vitamins (A, D, E, and K); nourish the skin, mucous membranes, and nerves; and serve as an anti-inflammatory. Healthy fat is utilized by the body in the form of essential fatty acids (EFAs).

Excessive fat intake, however, can contribute to a variety of illnesses, especially obesity and heart disease. Fat intake that is too low can also pose health risks. One of the keys to optimal health, then, is to make sure that you are getting an adequate supply of fats in your diet and that they are "good" fats, not fats that are harmful. These good fats, in the form of oils, remain liquid at room temperature.

The best food sources of healthy fats are the whole foods from which the oils are derived. These include foods such as nuts and seeds, soybeans, olives, and avocados. Healthy fats in the form of oils include olive, canola, flaxseed (do not use for cooking), and sesame. Essential fatty acids are found in two groups, the omega-3s and the omega-6s. Good sources of omega-3 include cold-water fish (salmon, sardines, tuna, sole), wild game, flaxseeds and flaxseed oil, canola oil, walnuts, pumpkin seeds, soybeans, fresh sea vegetables, and leafy greens. Good sources of omega-6 include vegetable oils, legumes, all nuts and seeds, most grains, breast milk, organ meats, lean meats, leafy greens, borage oil, evening primrose oil, and gooseberry and black currant oils.

Remember, getting the proper balance of essential fatty acids, through the NLEP and supplementation, can reduce overall inflammatory activity in the body and help relieve pain, even in your aching back.

Fiber

Fiber is one of the most overlooked components of a healthy diet, with the average American diet supplying only one-fourth to one-third of the amount necessary for optimal health. High fiber diets are associated with less coronary heart disease, lower cholesterol and triglyceride levels, lower blood pressure, lower incidence of cancer (especially colon and rectum), better control of diabetes, and lower incidences of diverticulitis, appendicitis, gall bladder disease, ulcerative colitis, and hernias. Lack of fiber is also the major cause of constipation and hemorrhoids.

Fiber includes the nondigestible substances in the foods that we eat. Good sources of fiber include fruits; the bran portion of whole grains, such as whole wheat, rolled oats, and brown rice; and raw and cooked green, yellow, and starchy vegetables such as spinach, romaine lettuce, squash, carrots, beans, and lentils. The goal is 25 to 35 grams of fiber per day.

THE NEW LIFE EATING PLAN HYPOALLERGENIC DIET

The first step in treating backache is to *remove* all inflammatory causes, since arthritis (an inflammatory condition) is a significant cause of chronic low back pain. Researchers at the National Public Health Institute in Helsinki, Finland, have recently discovered that people drinking four or more cups of *coffee* are twice as likely to develop arthritis than occasional drinkers. Anyone consuming eleven or more cups may be increasing their risk of arthritis by fifteen times—a significant risk in chronic backache. A relatively small proportion of people with arthritis have *food allergies* and sensitivities that cause joint inflammation. Dairy products, wheat, corn, citrus fruit, peanuts, and especially *nightshade plants,* including potatoes, peppers, eggplant, tomatoes, and tobacco, are the foods most often responsible for contributing to arthritis. The adverse effect from nightshades is not usually due to an allergic reaction but to a toxin called *solanine.* Eliminate nightshades from your diet for at least three months. The allergy elimination diet, as outlined below in the NLEP hypoallergenic Phase I diet, eliminates dairy, wheat, and any other repetitively eaten food for at least three weeks. This helps to determine if a food allergy is contributing to your back pain; gradually reintroducing them (one new food every three to four days) will reveal to you which specific foods, if any, are involved.

The next step in decreasing inflammation is to *remove* or *decrease* consumption of *most animal products* other than fish and healthy eggs, which will help to eliminate excess bad fats, calcium, mineral deposits, and acid from the joints.

The most effective way to permanently change your dietary habits is by following the New Life Eating Plan (NLEP) developed by Todd Nelson, N.D., a primary contributor to this book. He has for many years experienced excellent outcomes with his nutritional approach to treating many chronic illnesses, including back pain. (The NLEP has been used very successfully in the Arthritis and Asthma Survival Programs as well.) The NLEP is a nutrient-dense, hypoallergenic, low-yeast diet that is high in phytonutrients (e.g., berries, cherries, green and yellow vegetables), high in essential fatty acids, low in nightshades, and low in land-animal products. It helps in treating back pain by:

- Eliminating possible food allergens
- Stabilizing insulin levels—elevated insulin or low-insulin sensitivity can increase proinflammatory chemicals
- Correcting "leaky gut" and dysbiosis (an imbalance of the bacterial flora in the bowel) often resulting from long-term use of nonsteroidal anti-inflammatory drugs (NSAIDs). (Leaky gut contributes to inflammation of muscles and joints by recirculating large, undigested molecules that, in turn, trigger the inflammatory cascade of chemicals.)

The following is Phase I of the NLEP. For best results, the NLEP Phase I should be followed for a minimum of three months. Phase II of the NLEP, presented on page 126, expands your dietary choices to create and maintain a lifetime of exceptional eating.

NEW LIFE EATING PLAN: PHASE I
NUTRIENT-DENSE, HYPOALLERGENIC DIET
FOR BACKACHE

Vegetables

50 to 60 percent of total diet = 3 to 6 cups daily
High-water content vegetables
Raw or lightly steamed
Fresh, organic, clean

Steamed or stir-fried in water and spices:
> Most gentle (great for initial detoxification or cleansing diet)—zucchini, celery, green beans, spinach, parsley, crook-necked squash
> More difficult to digest—steamed broccoli, cabbage, bok choy, chard, kale, cauliflower, collard greens, mustard greens, beet greens

Raw:

> Baby greens, celery, carrots, cucumber, jicama, snow peas, sprouts, grated beets, red leaf lettuce, romaine lettuce, bib lettuce, green leaf lettuce, cauliflower, broccoli, radishes

Fruits

All fruits are acceptable except citrus—oranges, grapefruit, and the like (lemons are an exception)
Eat by themselves between meals, as snacks

Whole Grains

Sprouted or cooked like rice (see Grain Preparation Chart on page 210)
Organic, clean—available in bulk at health food stores
Only eat the nongluten grains—brown rice, millet, quinoa, amaranth
Rotate grains every four days
Tasty as breakfast cereals, in salads and soups, in casseroles and stir-fries (excellent for dinners)
Store away from light and heat in airtight containers
Combine with beans and legumes occasionally, if tolerated

Starchy Vegetables

Squashes
Avoid potatoes (they're nightshades)
If you want to try adding potatoes, use new red potatoes, sweet potatoes, or yams

Protein

Recommended—raw organic nuts (almonds, filberts, pecans) and seeds (sunflower, pumpkin, sesame, flax); raw organic nut butters (no peanuts); sprouted or soaked overnight or ground (12 nuts or handful of seeds = 1 serving)
Deep-water ocean fish (perch, salmon, halibut, orange roughy, sole, cod); farm-fresh fertile eggs, free of chemical additives
Ultra Clear (from Metagenics) beverages, under a physician's supervision

Soy—Tofu, soy yogurt, soy milk, tempeh
Minimize organic red meat, poultry, lamb
For vegetarians: bean and grain combinations are recommended
Protein powders—whey, soy, or rice-based

Flaxseed Oil

Do not heat or cook with flaxseed oil
1 to 2 tablespoons daily or 2 capsules two times daily with food
On grains or vegetables
With protein meals
As a salad dressing
Keep refrigerated and away from light
Use within 6 weeks of opening

Other Oils

Extra virgin olive oil—in salads, stir-fries, cooking
    Canola oil—in baking

Pure Water

Eight 8-oz. glasses (or ½ oz. per lb. of body weight) daily between meals (allow only 2 to 4 oz. with a meal)

Beverages

Fresh carrot, celery, or beet juice, or green drink, diluted 30 to 50 percent
Fresh fruit juices (not citrus), diluted 70 percent
Herb teas (not citrus)

MENU SUGGESTIONS FOR A NUTRIENT-DENSE, HYPOALLERGENIC DIET

Breakfast Suggestions

Nongluten whole grain porridge (recipe available at health food store)
Nongluten whole grain hot cereal (recipe available at health food store)

Grain Preparation Chart

Grain*	Grain Family	Gluten	Appearance (dry)	Uses
Amaranth	Amaranthus	No	Tiny, round, light-colored, speckled with black grain	In porridge, pancakes, vegetable dishes; ground as flour; used in baking
Barley	Cereal grass	Yes	Oblong, light-colored with a lengthwise "crease"	In salads, vegetable dishes, soups; ground as flour
Buckwheat	Sorrel	No	Groats—golden green, triangular-shaped; kasha—toasted groats, golden brown	In salads, vegetable dishes; ground as flour
Corn	Cereal grass	No	Polenta—coarsely stone-ground corn meal, yellow and brown	In porridge, cornbread, hominy, tortillas
Millet	Cereal grass	No	Small, round, lemon-tasting, yellow color	In salads, vegetable dishes, puddings, porridge
Oats	Cereal grass	Yes	Groats—long, slender, flake light brown	In porridge, salads; ground as flour
Quinoa	Goosefoot	No	White/brown, small discs	In salads, vegetable dishes
Rice	Cereal grass	No	Oblong, light-colored varieties	In salads, vegetable dishes, puddings; ground as flour
Rye	Cereal grass	Yes	Oblong, slender, gray/brown color	Sprouting, in salads, vegetable dishes, bread
Triticale	Cereal grass	Yes	Large, plump red/brown	Sprouting, in salads; ground as flour
Wheat	Cereal grass	Yes	Soft wheat—plump, oblong, slight brown color; hard wheat—small, oblong, brown	Sprouting, in salads, vegetable dishes; ground as flour

*For each grain, quantity is 1 cup.

Water	Cook	Yield	Comments
2 cups	20 min	1 cup	Very high in protein; slightly sticky texture.
3 cups	1 hr 15 min	3½ cups	Always barley "pot" barley, not refined "pearl."
2 cups	15–20 min	2½ cups	Chewy or soft, depending on the amount of water used.
4 cups	25 min	3 cups	Look for "stone ground" to avoid rancid oils.
3 cups	30–45 min	3½ cups	If bitter in taste, strain off initial cooking water and add new boiling water.
1½ cups	30 min	2½ cups	Large flake oatmeal is processed; occasional use is fine.
2 cups	15 min	3 cups	Pronounced "keen-wa"; very high in protein.
2 cups	45 min	3 cups	Many varieties; try short, or long grains; buy organic.
3 cups	1 hour	2½ cups	Stronger, heartier flavor than wheat with less gluten.
3 cups	30–60 min	2⅔ cups	Cross between rye and wheat.
3 cups	2 hrs	2⅔ cups	Bulgur, cracked wheat, and couscous are processed; use occasionally.

Note: If grains are presoaked, drain the soaking water, decrease cooking water by ½ cup, and decrease cooking time by 5 to 15 minutes.

111

Mochi waffle
½ baked acorn squash
Nut butters
Baked sweet potatoes
12 raw almonds, walnuts, filberts, pecans, or pine nuts
Small handful of raw sunflower seeds or pumpkin seeds
Ground raw sesame or flaxseeds sprinkled on hot cereal
Nut butter or nut milk
Steamed vegetables
Eggs and vegetables—omelette or basted with steamed veggies
Protein Smoothie: Blend together 4 oz. plain soy milk, 4 oz.
    water, soy or rice protein powder, ½ to 1 cup organic berries
    or cherries, ice cubes

Lunch Suggestions *(Protein/vegetable combinations)*

Fresh green salad with raw nuts or seeds
Fresh green salad with turkey, fish, lamb, beef, or chicken
Fresh green salad with sprouted beans or cooked beans
Steamed vegetables sprinkled with ground-up raw nuts or seeds
Steamed vegetables and an animal protein
Steamed vegetables or salad and bean, lentil, or pea soup
Vegetable and nut stir-fry (no rice)
Vegetable and animal protein stir-fry (no rice)
Fresh tuna salad with no mayonnaise
Vegetable and animal protein soup
Vegetable and bean soup
Vegetable soup or stew
Fresh vegetable sticks and nut butter for dip
Fresh vegetables and hummus for dip
Steamed asparagus wrapped in thinly sliced turkey breast
Turkey or chicken drumsticks and vegetables

Dinner Suggestions *(Complex carbohydrate/vegetable combinations; protein foods may also be added)*

Vegetable and nongluten whole grain casserole
Vegetable and nongluten whole grain salad

Vegetable and nongluten whole grain soup
Vegetable nori rolls with no mustard
Steamed vegetables or green salad with new red potatoes
Vegetables and baked squash or sweet potatoes
Vegetables with beans and rice
Vegetable stir-fry with a nongluten whole grain
Nongluten pasta salad
Nongluten pasta with dairy-free pesto sauce and vegetables
Dairy-free new red potato salad with vegetables
Vegetable sandwich on a nongluten whole grain bread★

Beverages

Herbal teas, noncitrus
Fresh, organic vegetable juice diluted 50 percent
Pure water
Fresh grated ginger-root tea

Flavorings

Flaxseed oil for salad dressings or in place of butter on steamed
    vegetables or cooked grains
Cold-pressed olive oil or sesame oil (Omega Nutrition)
Braggs Liquid Aminos
Fresh lemon or lime in dressings or on steamed vegetables
Fresh herbs—cilantro, mint, basil, dill, parsley, or rosemary to
    flavor salads and grains
Fresh spices (avoid salt and black pepper)
Use ghee instead of margarine or butter
Garlic (great for candida diets)
Ginger root
Nut butters for sauces and dressings

Allergy–Free Treats

Fresh organic fruit
Organic vegetable sticks

★Sauce and dressing recipes included on page 117.

Raw organic almonds, walnuts, filberts, pine nuts, sunflower
   seeds, pumpkin seeds
Rye crackers with raw nut butters
Smoothies
Nut milks or nut cheeses
Fresh juices (dilute 1:1 with water)
Juice popsicles
Frozen fruit popsicles
Applesauce or other fruit sauce
Baked apples
Steamed fruit
Fruit salad
Agar-agar and fruit juice mixed
Rice or millet pudding
Nongluten or whole grain muffins
Nongluten or whole grain pasta
Carrot, raisin, apple, or celery salad
Hummus
Leftovers
Nori roll

Recipes for a Nutrient-Dense, Hypoallergenic Diet

(For additional recipes, refer to the cookbook *Vital Abundance*
by Karen Falbo.)

Breakfast Recipes

WHOLE GRAIN PORRIDGE

Use leftover (already cooked) nongluten grains—brown rice,
millet, amaranth, or quinoa. Place the cold grain in the blender
with water, juice, rice milk, or nut milk. The amount of liquid
will determine how thick the porridge will be. Blend together
to desired consistency. Heat the porridge. Add pure maple syrup
and flaxseed oil to taste. Be creative and try other flavorings,
such as cinnamon, almond butter, banana, ground flaxseeds,
apple sauce, or almond slivers. No two porridges are alike. (For
candida diets, do not include fruit or sweeteners unless advised
otherwise.)

Whole Grain Hot Cereal

If you like Cream of Wheat, then try "cream of millet," "cream of amaranth," or "cream of quinoa." Pick any non-gluten grain and grind up ½ cup in a coffee grinder.

Add the grain very gradually to 1½ cups boiling water or apple juice, stirring constantly. Simmer for 5 minutes. Top it off with maple syrup, nut milk, and flax oil. Also try nuts and seeds, cinnamon, applesauce, or banana slices. It's quick, easy, and yummy! (For candida diets, do not add fruit or sweeteners unless advised otherwise.)

Nut Milk

Place ½ cup raw almonds, sunflower seeds, or sesame seeds, 1 tablespoon maple syrup or honey (optional), and 2 cups water in the blender. Blend until smooth and creamy. Strain milk through a cheesecloth. Flavor with cinnamon or pure vanilla. It's delicious hot or cold and a great milk substitute for baking.

Sprouted Grains

Soak a nongluten grain for 12 to 24 hours, rinsing twice daily until a tiny ¼-inch sprout begins to appear. At this point, spread the sprouts out on a towel and allow them to dry for 1 to 4 hours. Do not allow them to wither and harden. Place in refrigerator, and they will last 3 to 10 days. To serve, warm the sprouts very carefully in a pan with melted butter or soak in hot tap water for a minute or so. Eat them for breakfast or in place of cooked grains at other meals. Sprouts are high in fiber, the enzymes in the grains have not been destroyed by heat, and they are often less allergenic than cooked grains.

Acorn Squash

Cut squash in half and steam facedown for 20 to 30 minutes. Set on oven dish and fill with 1 teaspoon butter and 1 teaspoon honey or maple syrup. Place in 350°F oven for 10 minutes. Also delicious with flaxseed oil, but do not add until after baking. (For candida diets, avoid maple syrup or honey.)

Lunch and/or Dinner Recipes

BIELER'S BROTH

Steam 2 medium-size zucchini, a handful of green beans, and 2 stalks celery until they are very soft. Place the vegetables and the steaming water in the blender and blend for 1 to 2 minutes until smooth. Add fresh parsley and serve hot.

VEGETABLE SOUP

In a large saucepan, sauté diced celery, carrot, zucchini, broccoli, cauliflower, cabbage, onion, and garlic in a little pure water. Cover with water and add 1 tablespoon oregano, 1 tablespoon basil, and cayenne to taste. Simmer for 30 minutes. Serve, then add Bragg's Liquid Aminos to taste. Also try this soup with diced new red potatoes or sweet potatoes.

SPLIT PEA SOUP

Dice and sauté carrots, celery, and onions. Boil 1 cup green split peas in ½ to 1 quart water. Add vegetables after 20 minutes. Add ¼ teaspoon thyme.

CLEAN CASSEROLE

Steam zucchini and celery for 5 minutes. Turn off burner, add a good portion of mung bean sprouts, and let sit for 5 minutes. Place ½ inch of cooked rice in bottom of buttered casserole dish. Pour vegetables on top of rice and sprinkle with sunflower seeds. Bake at 350°F for 20 minutes. Allow to cool slightly, then add 1 to 2 tablespoons ghee or flaxseed oil, and sprinkle with Bragg's Liquid Aminos.

CURRY RICE

Sauté mushrooms and onions in ghee. Add cooked brown rice, a little tamari, and 2 tablespoons curry powder. Garnish with fresh chopped parsley. Serve with sautéed vegetables and a side of raisins and/or coconut.

QUINOA SALAD

1 cup quinoa, rinsed 2 to 3 times, 1¾ cups pure water, ½ cup finely diced cucumber or 4 celery stems, finely diced green onion, ¼ cup finely diced fresh cilantro, ⅓ cup corn kernels, 3

tablespoons fresh lime juice, 2 tablespoons sesame oil, 2 table-spoons flaxseed oil, sea salt to taste, 1 teaspoon rice syrup or honey (optional).

Bring water to a boil in a 1-quart pot, then add quinoa. Reduce heat and simmer, covered, for 15 minutes, stirring occasionally until grain is tender. Remove from heat and let cool, uncovered. Toss cucumber, green onion, cilantro, and corn kernels with cooked quinoa. Combine the lime juice, oils, salt, cayenne, and honey, and add to quinoa. Stir thoroughly with a fork to coat the grains and vegetables.

VEGGIE SANDWICH
Pile high on nongluten bread any or all of the following: grated carrot, cucumber, green pepper, onion, sprouts, lettuce, avocado. Sprinkle with your favorite herbs and spices.

ROSE'S SAUCE
Mix together 1 to 2 tablespoons flaxseed oil, 1 to 2 tablespoons raw sesame tahini, 2 teaspoons Bragg's Liquid Aminos, and fresh lemon juice to taste. Top with steamed vegetables (cabbage, onion, zucchini, and red peppers make a great combination) and wild rice. Serve hot. This also makes a great salad dressing if you decrease the tahini and increase the lemon juice. Add your favorite herbs and spices.

NONDAIRY SALAD DRESSING

¾ cup	(180 ml)	Omega brand flaxseed oil
¼ cup	(60 ml)	apple cider vinegar
1 tsp	(5 ml)	Dijon mustard
1 tsp	(5 ml)	Bragg Liquid Aminos
3 to 5 cloves		garlic (crushed)
6 drops		Tabasco sauce
1 tbsp	(15 ml)	sweet basil
½ tsp	(2 ml)	tarragon
½ tsp	(2 ml)	oregano
1 tsp	(5 ml)	maple syrup (optional)
1 tbsp	(15 ml)	capers

Blend in blender or food processor. Store leftover dressing in the fridge. The dressing will keep for several days. Add extra garlic if you like!

SUGGESTIONS FOR IMPLEMENTING THE DIET

(1) After shopping, chop up and store vegetables in separate containers for quick and easy use in stir-fries, salads, soups, and snacks.

(2) Cook 2 to 3 grains at once at the beginning of the week for convenient use as hot breakfast cereals or for use in salads, stir-fries, soups, and casseroles. Cooked grains will last five or more days in the refrigerator and can be frozen as well.

(3) Prepare a couple of healthy sauces or dressings ahead of time for easy meals with already chopped vegetables and prepared grains.

(4) Prepare large meals with plenty of leftovers for easy lunches and snacks. Freeze leftovers for future meals.

(5) Use an electric slow cooker for soups, stews, chilis, and beans.

(6) When steaming vegetables, save vegetable stock for later use in sauces and soups. You can freeze the stock, too.

(7) Make or buy healthy muffins, breads, or crackers to complement a salad or steamed vegetables or to eat as a snack.

(8) Keep your kitchen stocked with staples and foods for your favorite recipes.

(9) Freeze fruit such as bananas, blueberries, and grapes for snacks or use in smoothies.

(10) Take a water bottle with you wherever you go.

(11) Keep healthy snacks in your car and at work so you have healthy foods available when you get hungry.

Weight reduction, which is also strongly recommended in treating backache, should naturally occur when the NLEP and an exercise program are consistently practiced.

VITAMINS AND MINERALS

Note: In this section most of the products I recommend are available in health food stores, but some are only available through Sinus Survival Services. You can refer to the "Product Index" on page 291 for information on how you can obtain them.

Calcium is a strong contributor to cartilage health and is helpful to maintain bone density. In addition, it is critical to keep muscle functioning optimally. Muscle spasm is much more common in people with depleted levels of calcium and magnesium. The recommended amount of calcium, in a MCHA (microcrystalline hydroxyapatite) form, is 400 to 600 mg, three times per day. Calcium Supreme is a high-quality (MCHA) calcium containing glucosamine.

Magnesium is critical in maintaining proper muscle relaxation and preventing muscle spasm. Taking an exceptional form of magnesium and calcium daily is your best nutritional insurance against muscle spasm. Take 500 mg of magnesium per day in a glycinate form and calcium, as mentioned above, in a dose of 1000 to 1200 mg daily helps prevent muscle spasms. Herbal Muscle Relief contains magnesium, calcium, valerian, and passionflower (see Herbs table).

A significant number of people with backache are suffering from arthritis in their spine. However, it is estimated that in 85 percent of the cases of low back pain, a definitive diagnosis is *not* determined. For this reason, it is recommended that, if you do not have a precise diagnosis, you should include the following *Arthritis Survival* regimen as part of the Backache Survival Program.

Glucosamine sulfate is a naturally occurring building block of the substances (both proteoglycans and collagen) that make up cartilage. It is primarily produced in the body; but, as a dietary supplement, it is revolutionizing the treatment of arthritis. It has proven to be capable of both regenerating cartilage and inhibiting cartilage-degrading enzymes, thereby *slowing or preventing continued deterioration, while relieving joint pain and improving mobility.*

Although glucosamine is not an anti-inflammatory, a multitude of studies (nearly three hundred, including twenty double-blind studies) have shown that it can also effectively relieve the pain of osteoarthritis as well as NSAIDs, and with little or no side effects. One eight-week study compared the effects of glucosamine to ibuprofen. While the ibuprofen seemed to be working a bit better during the first two weeks and its benefits remained stable after that, those taking glucosamine continued to improve gradually throughout the remainder of the eight weeks.

The use of glucosamine for treating arthritis was first reported by German physicians in 1969, and for many years it has been approved for this use in a number of European countries. American veterinarians have been using it successfully on dogs and horses. On March 14, 2000, the American Medical Association (AMA) issued a news release describing a meta-analysis, published in the *Journal of the American Medical Association* (*JAMA*), which concluded that glucosamine and chondroitin supplements may have moderate to large therapeutic effects on osteoarthritis of the knee and hip. One landmark study, in which biopsies of arthritic knees were taken before and after thirty days of glucosamine sulfate therapy, dispels the commonly held belief that arthritis is an irreversible disease. The results showed that the degenerating cartilage had been replaced by much healthier cartilage.

This supplement is considered safe, but it can occasionally produce heartburn and diarrhea. This is probably because it is a difficult substance to digest, which is why it should be taken with meals. This will usually minimize or prevent the possible upset stomach. When capsules are ingested this way, about 90 percent of the glucosamine is absorbed into your body. Glucosamine promotes the healing of joints rather than merely relieving symptoms, and as a result it may take two to four weeks for pain relief and four to eight weeks to experience maximum benefit. Faster results can be obtained by adding an NSAID during the first two weeks. It is available in most health food stores. The recommended therapeutic dosage is 1000 mg three times per day for twelve weeks, followed by a maintenance dosage of 500 mg three times per day with meals (or 750 mg two times per day). One study suggests that people taking a diuretic may need to take higher doses of glucosamine to get its full effect. There are no known drug interactions, but there is some concern for diabetics (from animal studies) that it may raise blood sugar levels. The highest quality brands of glucosamine sulfate that I am familiar with are available through Sinus Survival Services and Enzymatic Therapy. Glucosamine can often be found in combination with the mineral boron, which can also improve the symptoms of arthritis. The daily dosage of boron is 6 to 9 mg.

Chondroitin sulfate is another naturally occurring component of joint cartilage. The body uses glucosamine to help make chondroitin. Although not as numerous as for glucosamine, there are several impressive studies documenting the therapeutic benefits of chondroitin for arthritis. In 1998, the journal *Osteoarthritis and Cartilage* published three double-blind placebo-controlled studies that documented the effectiveness of chondroitin sulfate in treating arthritis. It is widely used in Europe, primarily in an injectable form—injected directly into arthritic joints. This form of chondroitin is not readily available in the United States. Like glucosamine, oral chondroitin sulfate can *significantly reduce the pain and slow the progressive deterioration of the joints* in people suffering with arthritis. As you've already learned, there is no conventional treatment for arthritis that protects the joints and prevents them from worsening. It helps provide the body with the building blocks it needs to repair itself, and it also is believed to inhibit the activity of the enzymes that break down cartilage. Chondroitin works slowly, with improvement usually noted after three months and progressing up to one year or more. It is usually taken in combination with glucosamine. The recommended dosage is 400 mg three times per day. I recommend Glucosamine Intensive Care as a high-quality joint supplement combining glucosamine and chondroitin sulfate. Since chondroitin is difficult to digest, it should be taken with meals and with digestive enzymes.

Digestive enzymes, such as *bromelain* (found in pineapple), *papain* (found in papaya), *chymotrypsin,* and *pancreatin,* should be taken along with glucosamine and chondroitin to improve their digestion and absorption, hence improving their benefits. The enzymes can also reduce lymph congestion, toxicity, and tissue inflammation. Raw food enzymes, such as those found in the Metagenics product SpectraZyme, have also been effective in reducing food allergen antigens in the gut, which might contribute to inflammation in the joints. The enzymes are readily available in most health food stores.

Essential fatty acids (EFAs) in the form of *omega-3* oils, EPA/DHA, from cold-water fish (salmon, sardines, and tuna) and *flaxseed oil* (contains almost twice as much omega-3 as do fish oils) have been shown to significantly improve the symptoms of many forms of pain, including back pain and arthritis, primarily by inhibiting the process of cartilage destruction and by directly reducing inflammatory chemicals. The most effective way to take omega-3 oils is in the form of EPA (eicosapentaenoic acid) in a dosage of up to 600 mg four times per day for twelve weeks, then reduce to three times per day; DHA (docosahexaenoic acid), up to 400 mg four times per day for two months, then reduce to three times per day; and flaxseed oil, 1 tablespoon two times per day with meals or three capsules three times per day with meals. There are many varieties of EFAs available in health food stores containing EPA and DHA. However, you'll need to check the amounts of each of the oils to be sure you're taking the proper dosage. Super Potency Essential Fatty Acids (available through Sinus Survival) provides the recommended dosage.

The *antioxidants* are substances that prevent oxidation of cell membranes and thereby prevent cell damage. They include the following:

- *Vitamin C*—1000 to 6000 mg per day, in an ascorbate form or ester C (essential for collagen synthesis and connective tissue repair)
- *Vitamin A* or beta-carotene—10,000 to 25,000 IU per day
- *Vitamin E*—400 to 800 IU per day (has a mild antiinflammatory effect and increases proteoglycans)

The federal government's Institute of Medicine's April 2000 guidelines on recommended daily dosages for vitamins suggests a maximum of 2000 mg per day of vitamin C. The primary risk mentioned for megadoses of vitamin C was diarrhea. Using an ascorbate form of C or ester C reduces the possibility of these adverse side effects, since they are much better tolerated in the bowel than ascorbic acid (the most common form of vitamin C). If diarrhea does occur, you can simply reduce the dosage. I personally have been taking an average of 6000 mg of vitamin C daily for the past fifteen years without any problems whatsoever. In fact, I'm healthier than I've ever been and so are most of my patients, the majority of whom also exceed the recommended maximum daily dose of vitamin C. Linus Pauling, the two-time Nobel Prize winner who did much of the original research on the therapeutic benefits of vitamin C, took 10,000 mg daily and died at the age of 93.

A *vitamin B complex* is recommended at 50 to 100 mg daily, but especially important for backache are vitamins B_1, B_6 (both at 50 mg daily), B_{12} (0.25 mg daily), and folic acid (400 mcg daily). These B vitamins can enhance pain relief if taken with NSAIDs, thereby reducing the dosage and the harmful side effects of these anti-inflammatory medications. Proanthocyanidin, as *grape seed extract,* in a dosage of 100 to 300 mg per day acts as a strong anti-inflammatory. Masquelier's OPC (the highest-strength grape seed) is available through Sinus Survival. Mixed *bioflavonoids,* including quercetin, 500 mg three times per day, are helpful in reducing inflammation and supporting connective tissue. AMNI makes an excellent bioflavonoid called Flavanall, which is available through holistic physicians.

Vitamins B_{12} and B_1 (thiamine) in an injectable form can be a highly effective treatment for sciatica. Injected into the gluteal muscles in a dosage of B_{12}, 1cc + B_1, ½ cc, it can be administered three to seven times during the first one to two weeks. If, after ten injections, there is no improvement, then it should be stopped.

Colchicine, a naturally occurring alkaloid used in the treatment of gout, has been well documented to be of value in treating chronically painful herniated discs. It is administered through a series of intravenous injections two to three times weekly for three to six weeks. The dosage is 1 to 2 mg of colchicine diluted with between 10 and 15 cc calcium gluconate, sodium salicylate, or saline. This treatment can sometimes result in dramatic success in relieving pain, apparently due to the anti-inflammatory effect of colchicine.

Probiotics (products that help to restore normal bacterial flora to the bowel), consisting of *Lactobacillus acidophilus* and *bifidobacterium,* are particularly helpful in cases of dysbiosis, candidiasis, and leaky gut. Low-grade bacterial infections such as *Klebsiella pneumoniae* and parasitic infections like *Blastocystis hominis* have been linked to an increase in arthritic pain, especially in ankylosing spondylitis, due to their associated toxicity in the joints. Probiotics are effective in combating these low-grade infections in addition to healing a leaky gut. The dosage is ½ teaspoon, or two capsules, three times per day, preferably on an empty stomach. Buy only refrigerated brands that clearly state an expiration date between one and ten months from the date the item is purchased.

HERBS AND SPICES

Acute Muscle Spasm

- **Valerian root extract**—The word "valerian" is taken from the Latin, *valere,* "to be well." It has been used to treat nervous tension since pre-Christian times and is a natural sedative, antispasmotic, and sleep inducer. The major constituents of the herb, valepotriates, are well researched to be sedative, anticonvulsive, and tranquilizing. Valerian, when combined with passionflower and calcium/magnesium, is a powerful combination for relieving muscle spasm. High-quality valerian root is contained in the product Herbal Muscle Relief and is available through Sinus Survival Services.
- **Passionflower**—Used since the seventeenth century, passionflower extract contains alkyloids and flavonoids that have been well researched to have a relaxant effect on the central

nervous system. Passionflower is both anti-spasmotic and anti-inflammatory. Passionflower is contained in Herbal Muscle Relief available through Sinus Survival Services.

Muscle and Joint Pain

- **Boswellia** (*Boswellia serrata*)—This gum resin found in certain trees in India has a strong analgesic effect. The boswellic acids also provide a wide range of anti-inflammatory functions, reduce joint swelling, and increase blood supply to the joints, thus promoting healing. It has been researched and used extensively in India as an Ayurvedic (traditional Indian medicine) treatment for arthritis. It can be combined with curcumin and bromelain. The dosage is 500 mg standardized to 70 percent boswellic acids, three to five times per day between meals. Herbal Joint Relief meets this standard and includes curcumin, ginger, and cayenne (available through Sinus Survival Services).
- **Curcumin** (*Curcuma longa*)—An extract of the common spice turmeric, it is an effective anti-inflammatory and antioxidant. It increases secretion of cortisol (the body's natural cortisone) and also sensitizes receptors for adrenal hormones, making these hormones more effective as anti-inflammatory agents. Curcumin also helps to prevent the release of leukotriene (a substance that causes inflammation) from white blood cells. The recommended dosage is 400 mg containing 95 percent curcuminoids three times per day between meals and combined with 1000 mg of bromelain.
- **Ginger** (*Zingiber officinale*)—That this spice acts as an anti-inflammatory and natural COX2 inhibitor is well supported by scientific studies. It is also a digestive aid that soothes and relaxes the intestinal tract. The dosage is 0.5 to 1 mg of powdered ginger daily or as a tea—1 grated teaspoon of fresh ginger in a cup of hot water two times per day. More simply, you may take a standardized extract of ginger (at 5 percent or more gingerol) combined with 500 to 1000 mg of mixed bioflavonoids, or include it in your diet.
- **Cayenne** (*capsaicin*)—This spice is available as an OTC oint-

ment or cream for analgesia (blocks substance P, present in arthritic joints) and for increasing circulation to the joint. Cayenne ointment should be rubbed into the low back for relief of muscle pain or into the skin of the affected joints three to four times per day for at least a week. It is also available as a capsule, with a dosage of 500 mg three times per day.

- **Eucalyptus oil**—This oil contains ingredients that help to relax tight muscles and has been used for centuries by the Aborigines for treating backache. I've used and recommend to patients the same highly medicinal eucalyptus oil imported from Australia by Sinus Survival Services, for treating both backache and sinusitis.

- **White willow bark** (*Salix alba*) or meadowsweet—This substance contains salicin, the same active ingredient found in aspirin, which makes it an effective analgesic, especially for acute pain. The dosage is a 4:1 standardized extract, ½ teaspoon of tincture or two capsules, 200 to 400 mg, three times per day between meals.

- **Sarapin** (*Sarracenia purpurea*) or North American pitcher plant—Used as a local anesthetic, it can be injected into multiple painful muscles and trigger points (see page 164); the effects can last for up to three weeks; dosage is from 2 to 15 cc.

The New Life Eating Plan: Phase II

Now that you have been on Phase I for three to six months, you are ready to expand your food choices. I hope you have been able to stick to Phase I very closely and are reaping the benefits of renewed vitality, less back pain, greater joint mobility, better digestion, and an enthusiastic commitment to your self-care. At this point, it is natural for you to desire more variety in your food choices. But be careful! Many people will experience great results from eating like this and then adopt the attitude, "I've been doing well, so now I can go back to some of the old foods that I love." In fact, you might be tempted to go overboard in the opposite direction. The worst that can happen is that you will start feeling pain in your joints again. This is simply your body wisely reminding you to get back to a healthy diet. Let's now look at a safe, gradual way to expand your choices, while continuing to minimize toxicity and allergic reactions, and to maximize nutrient density.

At this point in your Backache Survival Program, try allowing the following list of foods back into your diet. Allow them only one at a time every four to six days so that you can be more aware of symptoms and track any food reactions. Score your symptoms each day on the symptom chart. If your symptoms seem to increase within a 24- to 72-hour period and you haven't made any other significant dietary changes, then you are probably reacting to that new food and should continue to avoid it. If you are unsure, keep that food out of your diet for seven days and retest it.

Once you know that you tolerate a food, allow it on a rotational basis, which means once every three to five days. For example, if you have a wheat product on Monday, wait until Thursday to have it again so your body has a chance to clear any reactions it may have to it. This also helps you to prevent developing a reaction to that specific food.

FOODS TO TEST ROTATING BACK INTO YOUR DIET

(These are foods to generally deemphasize in the diet and are not required to be healthy. They should only be allowed back in if you enjoy them and you continue to feel well while eating them.)

Wheat
Corn
Beans and legumes (if not already eating them)
Cheese
Cultured dairy—nonfat yogurt or cottage cheese
Red meat—avoid pork products for the long term
Citrus fruits
Whole grain rye crackers
Higher glycemic foods—flour-based foods such as whole grain pasta, breads, pancakes, muffins, and starchier fruits and vegetables. Use *very* sparingly.

Small amounts of sweetener—Stevia is best, or honey, maple syrup, and brown rice syrup

---

Remember: It's what you do most of the time—day in and day out—with your diet that counts. Maintain a lot of variety so you won't get bored. Do the best you can. Your back will let you know if you need to do better.

NUTRITIONAL SUPPLEMENTS

I believe that you can, by taking some simple and inexpensive measures, extend your life and your years of well-being. My most important recommendation is that you take vitamins every day to optimum amounts, to supplement the vitamins you receive in your food.

LINUS PAULING, PH.D., *two-time Nobel Prize laureate,*
who lived a full and productive 93 years by following his own advice

Following the dietary recommendations outlined above is a vital first step in creating optimal health for yourself and your loved ones. Sadly, however, a healthy diet alone, even one that is rich with pure, organically grown foods, is no longer enough to ensure total physical well-being. Due to our unhealthy environment and the stresses of daily life, most of us also need to supplement our diets in some fashion. On a daily basis we are exposed to stress in the form of chemicals, emotions, and infections. Chemical stress may come from polluted air and water, food pesticides, insecticides, heavy metals, and even radioactive wastes. More than ever before, foreign chemicals can be found in our foods and environment. Many of these are commercially synthesized, but quite a few are naturally occurring as well. In 1989, the Kellogg Report stated that 1,000 newly synthesized compounds are introduced into our environment every year. That's the equivalent of three new chemicals per day. Currently, there are approximately 100,000 of these foreign chemicals, or *xenobiotics,* in the world. They include drugs, pesticides, industrial chemicals, food additives and preservatives, and environmental pollutants. As a result, it's very easy for toxic chemicals to find their way into our bodies via the air we breathe, the foods we eat, and the water we drink. We also ingest these chemicals whenever we use drugs (both medicinal and illicit), alcohol, or tobacco.

Compounding this problem is the fact that the soil in which our foods are grown is greatly depleted of the trace minerals needed to create and maintain health. Many of our foods are shipped, frozen, stored, and warehoused, reaching us weeks or months after being harvested. Degeneration of their nutrient value occurs at each stop. Cooking methods, such as boiling and frying, also contribute to nutrient loss once the food reaches our kitchens and restaurants. Moreover, the standard American diet has become increasingly devoid of nutrients and overburdened with empty calories and nonfood additives. Therefore, even though the body is marvelously designed to eliminate toxins, in today's environment it needs help in doing so.

Free Radicals and Antioxidants

One of the biggest threats to our health are free radicals, highly toxic molecules that play a causative role in many disease conditions, particularly degenerative disorders such as arthritis, heart disease, cancer, cataracts, macular degeneration, high blood pressure, emphysema, cirrhosis of the liver, ulcers, toxemia during pregnancy, and mental disorders. Free radicals, or oxidants, are very unstable and highly reactive molecules that contain one or more unpaired electrons. They try to capture electrons off other molecules to gain stability, a process known as "oxidation." They also increase susceptibility to infection and accelerate the aging process by damaging the cells.

Since free radicals are the primary agents of most cellular damage, minimizing their harmful effects is important. Antioxidants are substances that significantly delay or inhibit oxidation. They neutralize free radicals by supplying electrons. Fortunately, our bodies manufacture antioxidant enzymes within the cells to neutralize and protect against free radicals. Working in tandem with antioxidant nutrients supplied by our diet, such as vitamin A, carotenes, vitamin C, vitamin E, copper, manganese, selenium, and zinc, these enzymes maintain healthy cell function in a variety of ways. As a result, so long as there is an adequate supply of oxygen, water, antioxidant nutrients, and enzymes in the body, cell damage is kept to a minimum. But when our bodies become deficient in any one of these health-enhancing agents, the cells are overrun by free radicals and the antioxidant defenses become unable to maintain their protective shield. This occurs whenever the body's production of antioxidant enzymes and our intake of antioxidant nutrients fall below what is needed to maintain good health. Poor diet, physical and emotional stress, exposure to pollutants, and lack of sleep all contribute to this decline in enzyme production. Escaping such stressors altogether is practically impossible in today's fast-paced world, but help is available in the form of vitamins and other nutritional antioxidant supplements that can offer substantial help in preventing disease, especially arthritis, and maintaining proper immune function.

The following table contains recommended dosages for the most common antioxidant vitamins and minerals, all of which should be part of anyone's daily regimen for creating and maintaining optimal health. There are a number of multivitamin formulas on the market that contain the ingredients listed below, or you can take them separately. Use the higher dosages whenever you are exposed to higher levels of stress, diminished sleep, increased exposure to pollutants, and other sources of toxicity, or when you are not eating as well as you should be. Otherwise, take at least the minimum dose every day, preferably with your meals.

RECOMMENDED DAILY NUTRITIONAL SUPPLEMENTS

Vitamin C (as polyascorbate or ester C)—1000 to 2000 mg three times per day
Beta-carotene—25,000 IU one to two times per day
Vitamin E—400 IU one to two times per day
B-complex vitamins—50 to 100 mg of each B vitamin per day
Selenium—100 to 200 mcg per day
Zinc picolinate—20 to 40 mg per day

Calcium hydroxyapatite—1000 mg per day
Magnesium glycinate or aspartate—500 mg per day
Chromium polynicotinate (ChromeMate®)—200 mcg per day
Manganese—10 to 15 mg per day
Copper—2 mg per day

4. EXERCISE AND REST

EXERCISE

Exercise can be quite beneficial to the backache sufferer, but only if it's done properly. This means not exercising immediately following a back injury or strain. Stretching should be the focus of your exercise for the first two months or longer. You can begin with low-impact exercise, preferably walking slowly, as soon as you're able to do so. Start very slowly and build the duration and intensity *very* gradually. In addition to walking, the most effective low-impact options are yoga, water walking, swimming, and Pilates, followed by aqua aerobics, ballroom or other low-impact dancing, and cycling (preferably on a reclining bike at low pedal resistance, over level surfaces at first).

Yoga

From my own experience and that of several of my holistic medical colleagues, I believe that *yoga may be not only the most therapeutic exercise but also probably the single best self-care therapy for treating chronic low back pain.* I've also been impressed by the survey results from the book *Backache Relief* by Arthur Klein and Dava Sobel. Published in 1985, the survey asked the 492 respondents who had been treated for backache to evaluate their practitioners based on the extent of the relief they experienced following their treatment. Yoga instructors fared best, with 96 percent of the respondents experiencing moderate-to-dramatic long-term relief from back pain after practicing the yoga positions they'd been taught. The complete results of the survey are as follows:

Practitioner	Moderate to Dramatic Long-Term Relief (%)	Temporary Relief (%)
Yoga instructors	96	4
Psychiatrists	86	0
Physical therapists	65	8
Acupuncturists	36	32
Chiropractors	28	28
Osteopathic physicians	28	15
Neurosurgeons	26	8
Orthopedists	23	9
Family practitioners	20	14
Massage therapists	10	63
Neurologists	4	4

Yoga, a Sanskrit word meaning "to yoke," refers to a balanced practice of physical exercise, breathing, and meditation to unify body, mind, and spirit, making yoga one of the most effective and ancient forms of holistic self-care. The benefits of this five-thousand-year-old system of mind-body training to improve flexibility, strength, and concentration are well documented. The basis of yoga is the *breath,* a variant of abdominal or belly breathing. There are a number of yogic systems; *hatha yoga* is most well known in the West. Hatha yoga postures, or *asanas,* affect specific muscle groups and organs to impart physical strength and flexibility, as well as emotional and mental peace of mind.

A variety of hatha yoga forms are available. Initially it is preferable to receive instruction for the first two or three months, due to the subtleties involved in yoga practice that are not apparent without firsthand experience of its practice under the guidance of a qualified yoga instructor. However, if that isn't possible, then I will attempt to be your teacher. You should begin yoga or a daily stretching regimen *only after you have given your back a chance to rest and heal following an injury.* For someone with backache, the practice of yoga is too valuable for you not to at least give it a fair trial. After consulting with several yoga instructors as well as referring to the book *Healing Back Pain Nat-*

urally, written by my holistic medical colleague (also a yoga teacher) and friend Art Brownstein, M.D., I have identified a group of yoga poses that are highly effective in producing long-term relief for low back pain. Each one is a relatively simple stretch that can be performed on a yoga mat or on a carpeted floor. In yoga there is no such thing as perfection or competition. It is not a goal-oriented practice, nor is there the belief in "no pain, no gain." With all of the following stretches, try to listen to your body and do *not* push to the point of pain. As you practice them daily, your flexibility will gradually increase. By trying to achieve too much too quickly, you can slow your progress and possibly injure yourself. Hold each one for 5 breaths, or approximately 30 to 60 seconds while breathing abdominally and through your nose if possible. Repeat each position twice. If a particular stretch is meant to be done on both sides of your body, such as in Knee to Chest, then do each side twice. Commit to spending at least 20 minutes daily practicing the following ten yoga poses. Remember to *breathe*. With some of the poses—for example, Cat-Cow—you'll be instructed to coordinate your breath with the stretch. Yoga can be very relaxing as well as remarkably helpful for your back. Enjoy the process!

(1) *Knee to Chest.* This position gently stretches the muscles in the hips, buttocks, knees, hamstrings, and lower spine and strengthens abdominal muscles while keeping the spine in a protected position. There are two options for performing this stretch. They both begin the same way. Lying on your back, slowly bring one knee up to your chest, or as high as you can without experiencing pain. You can keep your opposite knee bent or straight, whichever feels better (with back pain, it's usually more comfortable bent). In position A, clasp your hands on your shin between your knee and your ankle. In position B, clasp your hands on your lower thigh just above the back of the knee. In both positions, on every exhalation, gently pull or squeeze your knee closer to your chest. On every inhalation, relax. Keep the knee flexed with both the pulling/squeezing and releasing. Continue this slow,

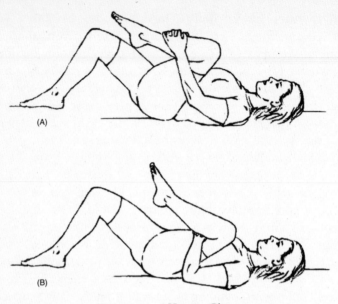

FIGURE 4.5 *Knee to Chest*

rhythmical breathing, while squeezing and relaxing. Feel the stretching in your hip joint, knee, and lower back. Repeat the same sequence with the opposite knee.

(2) *Supine Pelvic Tilt.* Lie on your back with your arms to your sides, palms down. Bend both knees, keeping your feet flat on the floor. With each inhalation, arch your low back while keeping your hips on the floor (A). This will create a space between your low back and the floor. Exhale and press your low back into the floor (B). Repeat this movement of tilting your pelvis back and forth at least 10 to 12 times.

(3) *Cat-Cow.* Place your hands directly under your shoulder joints, your knees under your hip joints, thighs and shins forming a right angle. Your feet are in alignment with your knees. Toes point straight, and soles of feet face upward. Your spine has the same curves as it did when you were lying on your back in exercise 2 above, but now you are turned over,

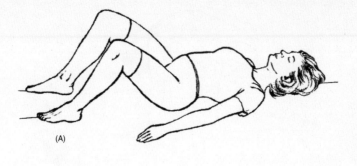

(A)

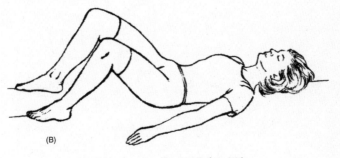

(B)

FIGURE 4.6   *Supine Pelvic Tilt*

and with this movement your spine will flex and extend as you tilt your pelvis back and forth. Another benefit of this position is that, by being on your hands and knees, all of the weight is off your back, allowing for a greater capacity to stretch and heighten mobility of the spine.

For the Cat Pose (A), inhale slowly, tuck your pelvis, drop your head, and round your back like an angry cat. Your hips (pelvis) are tucking and your spine is bending (flexing). This movement presses the air out of you, just like a bellows (exhale as you do it). You are also relaxing all the muscles in your head, neck, and shoulders as you do this stretch.

For the Cow Pose (B), tip your pelvis as you inhale slowly, lift your head, look up, and gently release the arch from your thoracic spine (midback), forming a concave curve. Move and breathe in a harmonious and relaxing

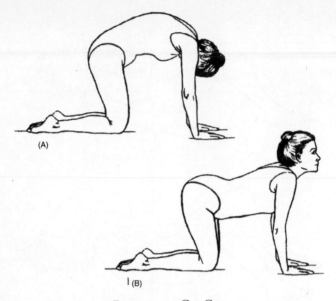

FIGURE 4.7   *Cat-Cow*

rhythm while doing 10 cycles initially, and gradually working up to 25 cycles.

(4) *Chair Forward Bend*. Sit in a chair with your knees wide
apart and your heels placed under your knees with your
toes pointed slightly inward. Use a chair with a firm seat
that allows your feet to be placed flat on the floor. Place
books under your feet if they're not flat on the floor. Be
sure your legs are parallel to each other, so that your shin-
bones provide support and you don't twist your knees. To
begin, slide your buttocks to the back of the chair and tilt
your trunk (from your waist up) forward to lean your elbows on your knees. Let your head hang forward so the
back of your neck is stretched. If this position is too uncomfortable or if you have high blood pressure, glaucoma,
or a detached retina, then maintain this pose for a few slow
abdominal breaths and go no further. If none of these pre-

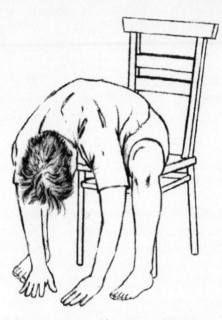

FIGURE 4.8   *Chair Forward Bend*

cautions applies to you, then tilt your trunk fully forward, letting your head and arms hang between your legs. If your hands don't touch the floor, then place them on books. Remain in this position and relax into it by tucking your chin slightly to stretch the back of your neck and soften the front of your neck as well. Hold this position for at least 20 to 30 seconds as long as you're not feeling pain. To come out of it, do not use your back muscles. Press your hands into the floor and begin moving up until your elbows rest on your knees, and then pause for several breaths. Then place your hands on your knees or on the seat of the chair, pushing your trunk upward while your head is still hanging forward. Straighten your head last, and then sit and breathe for another 10 to 20 seconds without moving.

(5) *Cobra*. Lie facedown on your belly. Place the palms of your hands on the floor in line with your chest, and your fin-

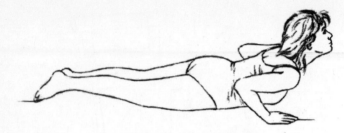

FIGURE 4.9   *Cobra*

gertips in line with your shoulders, with your elbows close
to your body, your feet together, and your forehead on the
floor. Slowly extend your head so that your chin first
touches the floor. Continue extending and lifting your
head off the floor while raising your upper body. Use only
your upper back muscles to lift (not your hands). Look up
as you extend your head and neck as far as you can without straining, while feeling a backward bending in your
spine. Come up only as high as is comfortable for you. Inhale as you do each progressive extension and raise your
upper body. To lower, reverse the order, lowering your
chest, then your chin, and then your forehead to the floor.
Repeat this cycle 5 times. Remember to breathe, and keep
only light pressure on your palms so that your back muscles are doing the work. Try to relax the muscles in your
buttocks as you maintain this position for as long as you
can without forcing or straining. After completing at least
5 cycles, turn your head to one side, close your eyes,
straighten and lower your arms to the floor, breathe, and
relax. In addition to stretching and strengthening the muscles that extend your spine as well as your abdominal muscles, this stretch also helps to open up the disc spaces.

(6) *Desk or Bridge Pose* (the counter pose of cobra). Lie on your
back and align your body as in exercise 2 above (Supine
Pelvic Tilt). This movement is very similar to the Cobra,
except that now, instead of your abdomen, your upper

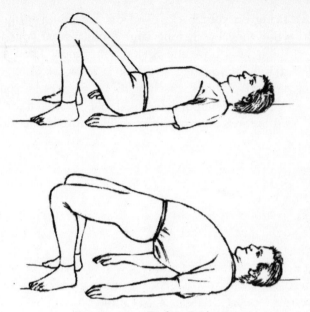

FIGURE 4.10 *Desk or Bridge Pose*

back becomes the base. Begin by exhaling and lifting your
hips just an inch off the floor while keeping your waistline
on the floor. If it's not uncomfortable for you to do so,
with each subsequent exhalation you can raise your pelvis
higher, but do so very slowly (about an inch with each out
breath). As you raise your pelvis, press down on your arms,
hands, and the inside edges of your feet. Keep your knees
and feet in alignment with your hip joints. Continue lifting up until you feel your lumbar spine (low back) beginning to arch.

(7) *Hamstring Stretch.* There are several methods for effectively
stretching the hamstrings. Located in the back of the thigh,
they are among the most powerful muscles in the body.
Every yoga instructor with whom I consulted emphasized
the importance of stretching the hamstrings in healing low
back pain. I'll present three options here.

(A) Lying on your back, bend one knee and bring it to your chest by clasping your hands behind your lower thigh just above the back of the knee. Then slowly straighten your leg at the knee joint, holding it in a vertical position, as close to 90 degrees as you can without forcing or straining. Hold the stretch for 30 to 60 seconds. It may be more comfortable to do this

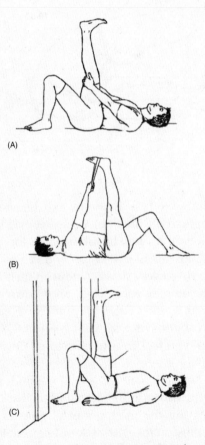

(A)

(B)

(C)

FIGURE 4.11   *Hamstring Stretch*

stretch if you bend the other knee while keeping that foot flat on the floor. To release this stretch you can slowly lower your leg to the floor, feeling its full weight as you lower it. Or if that's too uncomfortable, you can simply reverse the above stretch and bend your leg at the knee as you lower the leg and rest your foot on the floor. Repeat this stretch for the other leg.

(B) Begin this stretch just as you did in A above. However, instead of clasping your hands behind your thigh, place the center of a strap or belt on the ball of your foot before you gradually straighten your leg. Wrap the ends of the strap around your hands (ideally the strap should be approximately 6 to 8 feet in length) and hold for 30 to 60 seconds. The rest of this stretch is the same as A.

(C) This hamstring stretch uses a doorway or a wall to support your leg, keep your knee straight, and stretch the hamstring. It's very similar to A and B, but with this one you can rest your arms on the floor. I find it a little easier to do than the other two, and I'm able to hold the stretch much longer (3 to 5 minutes). With all three of these options, remember to stretch both legs.

(8) *Forward Bend.* Stand with feet parallel and about hip-width apart. Inhale while raising your arms up over your head with your palms facing each other. As you exhale, bend forward at the hips and gradually lower your hands toward the floor while slightly bending the knees (do not lock knees). Bend forward until you feel a gentle stretch in your hamstrings. Hold this position for 30 to 60 seconds while breathing.

(9) *Easy Back Twist.* Lie on your back with arms outstretched to the sides in a "T" position, with palms facing down. Bend your right knee and place your right foot on top of the left knee. Grasp your right knee with the left hand and gently draw the knee toward the floor on the left side of your body. Keep the right shoulder pressed to the floor, turn your head to the far right, and gaze at your right hand.

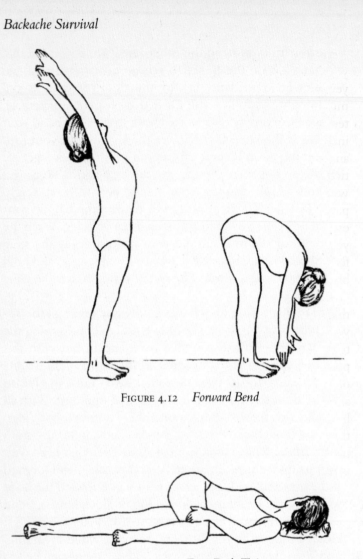

FIGURE 4.12 *Forward Bend*

FIGURE 4.13 *Easy Back Twist*

Hold for approximately 30 to 60 seconds, or 5 breaths. Release the knee and extend the leg and place it on the floor. Repeat the same sequence on the left side.

(10) *Relaxation Pose.* This should be the final position of your yoga session. It will help you to become more fully relaxed yet still conscious. It trains the body in stillness and the mind in alert quietness, and it teaches systematic release of tension throughout the entire body. With each inhalation, imagine that the breath is filling your chest, abdomen, back, and pelvis with cleansing or purifying air. With each exhalation, imagine that the breath is taking tension and toxins with it. Each in breath can illuminate and radiate in every part of your body that it enters. It is helpful and can be especially healing to see a bright white radiant light filling your low back with each breath. You should be very comfortable and warm in this pose, lying on a thick mat, a blanket (or under a blanket), or folded towels.

Begin by sitting on the floor with your knees bent and the soles of your feet on the floor. Place your hands behind your hips, palms down with your fingers under your buttocks. Lean back on your elbows, your chin in, chest expanded, and shoulders away from your ears. Rest the back of your pelvis on your hands. Press your feet to the floor and gently push your body backward, hips sliding over hands, until your whole back, pelvis to shoulders, rests on the floor. Your head then comes to the floor with the chin tucked and neck elongated. Slide your hands out from under your hips and turn palms up. Extend your arms out-

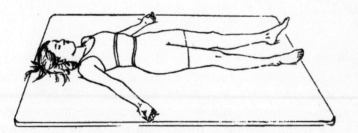

FIGURE 4.14 *Relaxation Pose*

ward about 15 degrees from your sides. Press your whole body downward into the floor—your feet, lower back, and the back of your neck and head. Feel your spine elongating. Exhale and relax. Extend first your right leg out on the floor, and then the left. Your feet, knees, and thighs turn outward.

Now turn your attention to yourself, while trying to detach from any noise, activity, and your thoughts. You are aware of all of them, but choose not to give them any of your attention. Try to focus on your breath as it flows in and out and feel the tension leave your body, from the crown of your head to the soles of your feet. Relax your tongue and your jaw muscles as your mouth opens slightly. Your arms and legs feel soft and heavy. Your hands and feet melt into the floor. Become very still and listen to the internal sounds of your body—the rhythmical beat of your heart, the breath flowing in and out.

Use the imagery described above and rest in this relaxed state for about 5 minutes before you slowly come out of the pose. Begin to stretch your fingers and toes wide apart. Roll onto your side, knees to chest, hands cushioning your head. After a few breaths, come up to a sitting position. Sit for a few minutes with legs and ankles crossed, spine straight, head centered, and hands on knees. Feel gratitude for the healing gift you've just given yourself. In addition to the therapeutic benefit to your back, the consistent practice of yoga, even for just 20 minutes a day, is one of the most beneficial health practices I've ever experienced—for body, mind, and soul.

Body Mechanics

Although body mechanics, improving posture, and workstation ergonomics are all services provided by *physical therapists* (see page 33), there are many things you can do on your own to improve your condition if you are more aware of how to better care for your back. Lifting heavy objects is one example. Lifting should be done by bending the hips and knees while keeping the back straight and the spine and shoulders over the hips. It is best to grab the object and hold it as close to your body as possible at your waist. Then stand up by straightening the knees and hips while keeping the spine straight. Follow this same procedure when putting down a heavy object—all the bending should be done with the hips and knees and not with the back. It is also very important when moving heavy objects to turn the entire body by turning the feet and legs, to avoid twisting the back. If the back is twisted while lifting, it is much more prone to injury.

It is better to push a heavy object rather than pull. Pulling is more likely to strain back muscles. Avoid shopping bags (with handles) for carrying groceries; carrying heavy things at arm's length places undue pressure on the low back. Instead, package groceries in a paper bag and carry it with both arms. When carrying a heavy object, it is always best to use both arms to distribute the weight evenly across your body and not heft it on one hip. When unloading a car trunk, it's recommended that you place a knee or foot on the bumper to improve your leverage.

As I mentioned in Chapter 2, prolonged sitting is a risk factor for low back pain, even if your posture is good. In a recent study, researchers measured muscle activity in fourteen locations on the back. They found that both slouching and sitting up straight stressed the back. To avoid this problem it's best to stand up and even take a brief walk every 15 to 20 minutes. If that's not possible, then shift your seating position, stretch, or do Kegel exercises. These are performed by contracting the PC muscle (pubococcygeus—the one you use to stop the flow of urine in midstream) for 5 seconds. Repeat these contractions several times. Regularly contracting the PC muscle has sexual benefits as well. It can help to prolong and intensify orgasm (it's essential in tantric sexual practice, which I discussed in *The Self-Care Guide to Holistic Medicine*), as well as massage the prostate. Isn't it interesting to see how much you can do for yourself without even getting out of your chair? Still, it's best for you to stand and walk briefly, since prolonged sitting is being repeatedly identified as a major risk factor for backache.

Strength Conditioning

Strength training is a vital part of any overall exercise program. It is also an integral component of the Backache Survival Program but should only be started after you have been practicing yoga or stretching for at least two months. Stretching alone will help considerably in creating a stronger back. You might recall that weak back muscles might have initially contributed to your problem, so you should begin a strengthening regimen very slowly while attentively listening to your body. If you do not, you run the risk of pushing too hard and possibly re-injuring your back. Stretching just before and after each strengthening exercise is very important.

The most effective exercises for strengthening the low back involve the leg muscles (especially the hamstrings), the gluteal muscles in the buttocks, the abdominal muscles, and the back muscles themselves. When legs are weak, too much stress is placed on the back, and pain not infrequently results. But when the legs are strong, back pain will usually diminish or disappear. The exercises most often recommended to backache sufferers for improving general strength of the leg muscles are walking, jogging, and cycling. Either or all of the hamstring stretches described in this Yoga section above should become a permanent part of your daily exercise regime. A simple exercise for strengthening the calves is to stand on your toes or sit on the edge of a stair and raise up onto your toes. Try to work up to 100 repetitions per day.

You can strengthen the gluteal muscles in your buttocks by lying on your back with your knees bent and gently squeezing your buttocks as tight as you can. This exercise can be repeated 100 times before you get out of bed every morning, and again in the evening before going to sleep. It is also very helpful if you are in severe pain and can't get off the floor or out of bed.

Strengthening the abdominal muscles can be a challenge because of the risk of re-injuring the low back. However, if you make your movements slow and smooth, avoiding jerky, rapid motions that can strain the back, you should have no problem. Sit-ups with knees bent (also called abdominal crunches) and leg lifts are both good for strengthening abdominal muscles. The leg lifts should be done one leg at a time, which is much safer for the back and can be performed on the floor or on your bed or a sofa with your legs dangling off the side. After several weeks of one leg, try doing both legs together. With both sit-ups and leg lifts, begin *very gradually* with 5 or fewer repetitions daily at the beginning, slowly building up to a maximum of no more than 35 to 50 repetitions per day. Focus on quality and smoothness of execution, not speed or quantity.

Yoga is the best method for strengthening the back muscles. Just by practicing the yogic stretches described above on a daily basis, you can improve the strength of your back muscles considerably.

Walking, swimming, and cycling are also helpful for strengthening back muscles. With *walking,* you'll want to increase your time, distance, and degree of difficulty (hills) slowly. Begin with 5 minutes a day and build up to at least 30 minutes, 3 to 6 days a week by adding 5 minutes to your walk each week.

Swimming has the advantage of having no weight on the spine, which reduces the risk of strain or injury while you are strengthening your back muscles. The kicking movements are especially helpful for building up the muscles in the lower spine, buttocks, hips, and legs. Treading water while doing a scissors kick or holding onto a wall or kickboard and doing either a crawl or frog kick are excellent ways to strengthen the muscles of the low back. You can vary your swimming stroke—freestyle, breast, back, or side—but be sure to focus on your kick, since that's the primary back strengthener. Remember not to push yourself or strain too hard and to stretch before and after your swim.

Stretching, especially the hamstrings, is also a requirement if you decide to *jog* as your method of strengthening your back. Jogging without stretching results in extremely tight leg and back muscles, which can trigger further back problems. Softer surfaces, such as grass, dirt, and sand, are less jarring and much easier on the spine. You shouldn't begin jogging until you're able to walk for at least 30 minutes a day without back discomfort. Start out at a very slow pace, 10 minutes every other day for two weeks. Stretch both before and after each jog and on your days off, focusing on the hamstrings. If you've had no pain during the first two weeks, you can increase to 20 minutes every other day with the same stretching instructions as above. After two more weeks you can increase to 30 minutes a day, 3 to 6 days a week. If you're experiencing back pain during, after, or the day following a jog, you'll have to make some adjustment to your regimen. Either reduce the time, intensity, distance, or frequency.

Remember that the key to success with the Backache Survival Program is to *listen to the messages your body is sending you every day, heighten your awareness of what you need, and use that information to learn to love, nurture, and heal your back.* If you ignore the pain, you run the risk of re-injuring your back. As you'll discover in Chapter 5, the physical pain may be reflecting a painful emotion that you're not expressing (or are not even aware of), and not simply a result of doing too much exercise, although that, too, may be a factor. If you attempt to swim or jog through the pain, you will have missed the opportunity to understand more about why you've been suffering with backache in the first place.

Cycling can also be an effective method for supporting the back by strengthening the leg muscles. The problem with cycling, however, is that most bikes, stationary or moving, require you to sit in a bent-over position, which places more stress on the back. In recent years, recumbent bikes, which eliminate this problem, have become more commonplace. Follow the same instructions for cycling as I've described for jogging. Begin gradually and work your way up to 30 to 40 minutes a day, 3 to 6 days a week. Stretching your hamstrings, especially, as well as doing the other yoga stretches on your cycling days, is essential.

This same stretching requirement along with listening to your body holds true for any back strengthening exercise. In addition to walking, swimming, jogging, and cycling, you can also participate in low-impact aerobics, calisthenics, and many sports and physical activities. These might include, among others, tennis, golf, skiing, hiking, or sailing. While engaged in any of these activities, it is important to be aware of your back and take it easy on yourself. The health benefits of participation in your favorite sport go far beyond simply the rehabilitation of your back. Dr. Art Brownstein, an accomplished athlete who suffered with back pain for fifteen years, writes in his book *Healing Back Pain Naturally:*

> You may not be able to do what it is you love now because of your back, but if you hold that goal in front of you, you are much more likely to be motivated to do the work that will take you back to it soon. When you do come back to your favorite sport after a long lay-off due to an injury, you will appreciate participating more than ever before. A spirit of gratitude will permeate your being and you will play with more grace and style. You will be smarter, wiser, and you will discover a deeper, inner aspect to the game that is more uplifting and personally enriching than the competitive thrill of winning.

He also recommends reading *The Way of the Peaceful Warrior* by Dan Millman. It is the true story of a college gymnast who recovered from a devastating injury and won an Olympic gold medal. I, too, found it to be a profoundly inspirational book and agree that it would be especially valuable for anyone needing some added motivation to heal his or her back.

The survey mentioned on page 131 highlighted yoga as the single most effective therapy for producing moderate to dramatic long-term improvement of backache. You are also aware that all of the strengthening exercises described above should be accompanied by stretching. I will also add that nearly everyone I know who has cured themselves of incapacitating back problems has maintained a lifelong practice of yoga or daily stretching exercises. Keep this information in mind as you read the following discussion of exercise and physical activity. I realize that your initial objective in reading this book is to be free of back pain. If you practice consistently for several months the exercises on the pages above, along with the other recommendations presented earlier in this chapter, you will have an excellent chance of achieving your goal. In addition, you might also want to try one of the professional care therapies beginning on page 162. However, I'd like to offer you another option, if you're interested in going further. It is possible to heal your back, that is, to be free of back pain, while also feeling more fully alive. This state of well-being encompasses a degree of physical, mental, emotional, spiritual, and social fitness you probably have never known. Your backache reflects an imbalance in your life that needs to be addressed before your back can be healed, even though you may be pain-free. This and the following two chapters are focused on healing your back as well as your life.

To go beyond a pain-free back to a state of optimal physical health, you must engage in a comprehensive exercise program—along with the healthy environment and diet that have been discussed earlier in this chapter. I recognize that for many of you exercise has in the past triggered back pain. But I also know that if you're willing to follow the exercise recommendations on the previous pages that are primarily focused on your back, while also expanding your program to include the following suggestions, you can learn to reap the full benefits of exercise without aggravating your back. The more complete the exercise regimen, the more it will affect your whole body. It should be started after you've practiced the back stretching and strengthening exercises for two to three months. And as with the previous exercises, remember to start slowly, but be persistent and allow your body to determine its own limits.

Regular exercise has the potential to contribute more to creating a condition of optimal health than any other health practice. Yet, in spite of exercise's many proven benefits, we are becoming an increasingly sedentary nation. This is especially true of our children, who are becoming fatter (25 percent are overweight), weaker, and slower than ever before.

Numerous studies show that sedentary people, on average,

don't live as long or enjoy as good health as those who get regular aerobic exercise in the form of brisk walking, jogging, swimming, cycling, rebounding, or similar workouts. In fact, some researchers now believe that lack of exercise may be a more significant risk factor for decreased life expectancy than the *combined* risks of cigarette smoking, high cholesterol, being overweight, and high blood pressure. Simply put, *being unfit means being unhealthy.*

The benefits of regular exercise and physical activity include lessening of tension and *decreased* "fight or flight" response, depression, anxiety, smoking, drug use, and incidence of heart disease and cancer; *increased* self-esteem, positive attitudes, joy, spontaneity, mental acuity, mental function, aerobic capacity, and enhanced energy; *increased* muscular strength and flexibility; and *improved* quality of sleep. Regular exercise also results in an increased muscle-to-fat ratio and increased longevity—people who are least fit have a mortality rate three and a half times that of those who are most fit.

Some of the more pronounced benefits of regular exercise occur with older women. A seven-year study conducted by the University of Minnesota School of Public Health tracked the physical activity levels of over 40,000 women, all of whom were postmenopausal and ranged in age from 55 to 69. The results showed that women who exercised at least four times a week at high intensity had up to a 30 percent lowered risk of early death compared to women in the same age group who were sedentary. But even infrequent exercisers among participants in the study (once per week) experienced reduced mortality rates.

In selecting an exercise program, choose a blend of activities that will increase *aerobic capacity, strength,* and *flexibility.* A regimen focused solely on strength conditioning, such as weight lifting, while providing strength, does little to increase aerobic capacity and can even diminish flexibility. Adding a stretching routine and an aerobic workout on alternate days will provide a much more effective exercise practice. In making your exercise choices, be aware of how it might affect your back. For instance, many people injure their backs while weight lifting, so I do not recommend that strengthening option for my patients with backache. I would also avoid the aerobic options of long-distance running or high-impact aerobics classes.

Aerobic Exercise

The word "aerobic" means "with oxygen." Aerobic exercise refers to prolonged exercise that requires extra oxygen to supply energy to the muscles. In general, aerobic activities cause moderate shortness of breath, perspiring, and doubling of the resting pulse rate. A few words of conversation should be possible at the height of activity; otherwise, the workout may in fact be too strenuous.

Aerobic exercise is based on maintaining your *target heart rate,* producing greater benefits to the cardiovascular system and providing more oxygen to the body than any other form of exercise. To determine what your target heart rate should be, use the following formula: 220 minus your age, multiplied by 60 to 85 percent. Keep in mind that 60 percent is considered low-intensity aerobic exercise, with 70 percent being moderate and 85 percent high intensity. For example, a 40-year-old's target heart rate is between 108 and 153 beats per minute. To accurately determine your pulse, use your index and middle finger to feel the pulse on the thumb side of your wrist or at your neck, just below the jaw. Using a watch with a second hand, count the number of beats in 60 seconds, which will give you your heart rate in beats per minute (or count for 15 seconds and multiply by four).

When you have attained your target heart rate—for the average person that should take about 5 to 10 minutes of exercising—try to maintain it for at least 20 minutes. It is also beneficial to cool down by working out at a slower heart rate and with less intensity for an additional 5 to 10 minutes before you end your session.

The most convenient forms of aerobic exercise involving the least amount of wear and tear on the body are brisk walking, hiking, swimming, rebounding (jumping on a mini-trampoline), and cycling. Cross-country skiing, if convenient, can also provide a very good aerobic workout. Jogging can also be effective, but to avoid injury (especially to your back) it is recommended that you stretch thoroughly before and after each run, use good running shoes and orthotics—if indicated—and supplement with vitamin C, calcium, and collagen to strengthen your bones, cartilage, muscles, and tendons. Treadmills, rowing machines, stair climbers, stationary bikes (the recumbent bikes are best), and cross-country ski machines also offer an opportunity for excellent indoor aerobics, as do low-impact aerobics classes. Racquetball, handball, badminton, and singles tennis provide good aerobic workouts as well.

The keys to a successful aerobic routine are consistency and comfort. Aerobic conditioning does not have to entail a great deal of time, nor should it be painful. Find an activity that you can enjoy and keep it fun. Remember, too, that low to moderate aerobic exercise for 45 minutes is just as beneficial as high intensity for 20 minutes. *Do not begin any aerobic activity in the heat of an emotional crisis, especially intense anger.* Wait at least 15 to 20 minutes to avoid the risk of heart attack or arrhythmias that can be triggered under such circumstances. In addition, make sure your aerobic exercise precedes meals by at least 30 minutes or follows them by at least 2½ hours, in order to avoid indigestion.

Exercise outdoors, if you live or work where it is convenient and safe to do so (specifically with regard to automobile traffic and outdoor air quality and temperature). Remember, too, that softer surfaces, such as grass, dirt, and sand, are more gentle on your back. When you exercise, you may increase your intake of air by as much as ten times your level at rest. The combination of fresh air and sunshine provides greater health benefits than indoor exercise. For chronic respiratory disease sufferers and for those practicing respiratory preventive medicine, air quality is a critical factor in determining where and when to exercise. Ozone, one of the most harmful air pollutants, is created by the combination of nitrogen oxides, hydrocarbons, and sunlight. A bright sunny day in the downtown area of most large cities will produce high concentrations of ozone. The EPA considers air unhealthy when ozone levels top 0.125 parts per million. However, in a study conducted by New York University's Morton Lippman, M.D., thirty healthy adults showed decreases in lung capacity during 30 minutes of exercise at ozone levels below the federal limit.

I suggest scheduling exercise around the rise and fall of pollution levels. In the summer, ozone builds up during the morning, reaches its maximum late in the afternoon, and then ebbs in the evening. In the winter, ozone isn't such a problem, but cold night air can trap a layer of carbon monoxide, nitrogen dioxide, sulfur dioxide, and particulates that can linger into the early morning. A good general practice is to do outdoor exercise in the morning during the summer and in the early evening during the winter.

If you are used to walking, biking, or jogging along main roads, lung specialists recommend that you stay away from these high-traffic areas during rush hour. Avoid waiting beside stop signs or stoplights, where carbon monoxide builds up. Henry Going, M.D., a UCLA pulmonologist, says, "I've seen guys jogging in place next to cars at stoplights. You might as well smoke a cigarette." On windy days, pollution disperses quickly the further you move away from the road. On calm days, it can extend about sixty feet from either side of the road.

If all of these concerns pose too great an obstacle or if you live in a highly polluted city, it's a good idea to head indoors for aerobic exercise. Remember that mouth breathing during exercise bypasses the nose and sinuses, your body's natural air filter, so try to remember to *breathe through your nose.* Air pollution can more easily aggravate asthma and chronic bronchitis during exercise. Ozone levels in most homes, gyms, and pools are about half that of the outdoors—even less with a good air-conditioning system.

William S. Silvers, M.D., a Denver allergist with whom I collaborated on the first Sinus Survival study, has found that many patients with respiratory difficulties who exercise regularly and follow this with a wet steam exposure experience improved breathing, increased mucus flow and expectoration, and less nasal and throat congestion. He recommends that, following your 20 to 30 minutes of aerobic exercise, and after your heart rate has dropped to its pre-exercise level, you expose yourself to wet steam for 5 to 10 minutes. This can be done in a steam room at a health club, the bathroom of your home, with a steam inhaler, or by standing over a boiling pot of water with a towel over your head. You should do nasal/chest breathing, which is best performed by taking a deep, slow inhalation through your nose and then breathing out from your chest. Do this as many days as you can, whether you exercise indoors or outdoors.

Moderate exercise is less strenuous than aerobic but is still beneficial. In a research project at the University of Minnesota School of Public Health, "moderate exercise" was defined as rapid walking, bowling, gardening, yard work, home repairs, dancing, and home exercise, conducted for about an hour daily. A treadmill test determined that those who got this much leisure-time exercise had healthier hearts than those who got less or none. There was no added benefit in doing more than an hour's worth of physical activity. Robert E. Thayer, Ph.D., a professor of psychology at California State University, Long Beach, has found that brisk walks only 10 minutes long can increase people's feelings of energy (sometimes for several hours), reduce tension, and make personal problems appear less serious. Not only does it nourish mind and body, but *walking is also by far the easiest, safest, and least expensive (you need only comfortable shoes) form of exercise.* Briskly walking 2 miles at 3.5 to 4 miles per hour (or 17 to 15 minutes per mile) burns nearly as many calories as running at a moderate pace and confers similar fitness benefits. By swinging your arms, you'll burn 5 to 10 percent more calories and get an upper-body workout as well.

Strength Conditioning

As you learned above, building and maintaining muscle strength are essential components of your overall exercise program. Strength conditioning falls under the following three categories:

- *Strengthening without aids*—includes calisthenics such as sit-ups, push-ups, jumping jacks, yoga, and swimming
- *Strengthening with aids*—includes chin-ups, dips, weight lifting, and training on weight machines
- *Strengthening with aerobics*—involves various forms of interval training that can be done running, bicycling, jumping rope, circuit training with weight machines, and working out on a heavy bag.

The goal of interval training is to work intensively, reaching your maximum heart level for a short interval, then lowering the level of activity to recover. Repeating this process while maintaining your heart rate in its target zone reduces recovery time, strengthens various muscle groups, and conditions the cardiovascular system.

Weight training is perhaps the most popular form of strength-conditioning exercise. To design a weight program to meet your specific needs (especially if you have a history of low back pain), consult with a personal trainer, who will most likely advise you to work out two to three times a week. (If you have a history of backache, I would recommend weight training only with great caution.) It isn't necessary to lift a lot of weight to build and tone muscle. If muscle tone and definition are your goals, best results will be achieved using less weight and more repetitions. To build mass, increase the amount of weight you use and do fewer repetitions. Remember to breathe *out* and be sure not to hold your breath during weight training as you exert effort. For free-weight exercises it is advisable to work with a spotter. Also, wear a weight belt to help keep your spine properly aligned. If you are unable to begin weight training with a personal trainer, I would not recommend doing this on your own.

Increasing Flexibility

The final component of a good exercise program addresses flexibility. This includes stretching exercises, yoga, tai chi, and the Feldenkrais Method. Exercise that promotes flexibility also significantly contributes to strength and function by allowing the body's muscle groups to perform at maximum efficiency. Lack of flexibility can severely inhibit physical performance, increase the potential for injury, and compromise posture. Muscles exist in a state of static tension wherein contrasting sets of muscles exert similar force to create a state of balance. When muscles become weak or inflexible, this balance is disrupted, resulting in reduced function or postural misalignment. Additional benefits of muscle flexibility include improved circulation, enhanced suppleness of connective tissue (tendons and ligaments), decreased risk of injury, and greater body awareness.

Stretching exercises Some form of stretching is recommended before and after both aerobic and strengthening workouts. Before you begin stretching, do 5 minutes of movement to warm up your muscles and body core. This will enhance your circulation and make stretching easier. Never stretch to the point of pain. Ideally, you should feel a tension in the affected muscle or muscle group that you are working. As you do, breathe into the stretch to elongate and relax the muscle group as you hold the posture for 20 to 30 seconds. Repeat each stretch at least twice. You should notice that your range increases on the second and third repetition. A few minutes of daily stretching will noticeably improve your well-being over time. (Yoga has already been discussed in detail, beginning on page 131.)

Tai chi Sometimes referred to as "meditation in motion," tai chi or tai chi chuan, like yoga, is thousands of years old. It involves slow-motion movements integrated with focused belly breathing and visualization and is practiced daily by tens of millions of people in mainland China. The goal of tai chi is to move *qi* ("chee"), or *vital life force energy,* along the various meridians, or energetic pathways, of the body's various organ systems. According to traditional Chinese medicine, when the flow of *qi* is balanced and unobstructed, both blood flow and lymph flow are enhanced, and the body's neurological impulses function at optimal capacity. The result is greater vitality, resistance to disease, better balance, stimulation of the "relaxation response," increased oxygenation of the blood, deeper sleep, and increased mind-body awareness. Although not as well known as yoga in this country, tai chi is rapidly gaining in popularity, and tai chi instructors can be found in most metropolitan areas. After being taught the basic movements of tai chi, you can practice them almost anywhere to instill a centeredness and sense of calm and to alleviate stress. It can also be quite helpful for someone with backache.

SLEEP AND RELAXATION

While diet, the use of supplements, and exercise can all benefit your back and your overall physical health and improve immune function, perhaps the most powerful and overlooked key to overall well-being is sleep. The average person requires between 8 and 9 hours of uninterrupted sleep, yet in the United States we average between 6 and 8 hours, with an estimated 50 million Americans suffering from insomnia.

Lack of sleep and its resulting depression of the immune system can be a factor in many chronic health conditions and is one of the most common causes of colds and sinus infections. Additional sleep is therefore an essential component in the holistic treatment of such conditions. Besides lowered immune function, sleep deprivation can also cause a decrease in productivity, creativity, and job performance and can affect mood and mental alertness. In cases of insomnia, most incidents of sleep deprivation are due to a specific stress-producing event. While stress-induced insomnia is usually temporary, it may persist well beyond the precipitating event to become a chronic problem. Overstimulation of the nervous system (especially from caffeine, salt, or sugar) and simply the fear that you can't fall asleep are other common causes.

Researchers have identified two types of sleep—*heavy* and *light*. During heavier, or nonrapid-eye-movement (NREM) sleep, your body's self-repair and healing mechanisms are revitalized, enabling your body to repair itself. During lighter, rapid-eye-movement (REM) sleep, you dream more, releasing stress and tension. (For more on dreams, see Chapter 5.)

Conventional medicine commonly prescribes sleeping pills for insomnia and other sleep disorders, but, as with almost all medications, there are unpleasant side effects to contend with, as well as the risk of developing dependency. A more holistic approach to ensuring adequate sleep begins with establishing a regular bedtime every night so that you can begin to reattune yourself to nature's rhythms. By not awakening to an alarm clock, you allow your body to get the amount of sleep that it requires. Try going to sleep earlier if you find you still need an alarm clock.

Many insomniacs (those that awaken in the middle of the night and can't fall back to sleep) have developed the habit of "clock watching" during the night when they wake up. They typically have an alarm clock with bright red digits glaring at them in the darkness. They actually may have trained their unconscious mind to *look for* those preprogrammed times. The silent message that they consistently hear (especially before going to bed) is "I wake up every night at ___ a.m." As this pattern of awakening too early continues, they are literally creating the expectation to awaken at their designated time, and their hormones and nervous system follow their explicit instructions. An effective method for breaking this habit is to never check the time, turn the clock around so that it's facing away from them, or turn it off! This practice, developed by Dr. Todd Nelson, has worked well for many of his patients who were able to stop their clock watching and, as a result, end their insomnia.

According to Ayurvedic medicine (the traditional medicine of India), the circadian rhythm, caused by the Earth rotating on its axis every 24 hours, has a counterpart in the human body.

Modern science has confirmed that many neurological and endocrine functions follow this circadian rhythm, including the sleep-wakefulness cycle. Ayurveda teaches that the ideal bedtime for the deepest sleep and for being in sync with this natural rhythm is 10 p.m. Unfortunately, most people with insomnia dread bedtime and go to bed later, when sleep tends to be somewhat lighter and more active. Ayurveda also states that 8 hours of sleep beginning at 9:30 p.m. is twice as restful as 8 hours beginning at 2 a.m. It is also important in resetting your biological clock to get up early and at the same time every day, regardless of when you go to bed. Establishing an early wake-up time (6 or 7 a.m.) is essential for overcoming insomnia. You'll eventually begin to feel sleepier earlier in the evening, and even if you aren't actually sleeping by 10 p.m., you'll benefit just by resting in bed at that hour.

Other natural remedies include:

- Vitamin B complex, 50 to 100 mg daily with meals; the best food sources of the B vitamins are liver, whole grains, wheat germ, tuna, walnuts, peanuts, bananas, sunflower seeds, and blackstrap molasses
- Niacinamide (vitamin B_3) up to 1 gram (1000 mg) at bedtime, for people who have trouble staying asleep, not falling asleep
- Calcium and magnesium, 500 to 1000 mg of each within 45 minutes of bedtime
- Chamomile, passionflower, hops, skullcap, and especially valerian herbs; they are natural sedatives that do not alter the quality of sleep the way prescription and over-the-counter drugs do; they can all be taken as a tea, while valerian and passionflower are available in stronger dosages in a tincture form
- Kava kava is another useful herb for both anxiety and insomnia; recommended dosage for sleep is two to three capsules (60 to 75 mg per capsule) taken 1 hour before bedtime
- Tryptophan, 3 to 5 grams taken 45 minutes before retiring, and at least 1½ hours after eating protein; adding B_6 to the tryptophan along with fruit juice can improve results; available by prescription only

- 5-hydroxytryptophan (5-HTP), 100 to 250 mg before bed
- Melatonin, a hormone produced by the pineal gland in response to darkness—most effective for difficulty falling asleep; recommended dosage ranges from 1 to 4 mg, 30 to 60 minutes before bed; can also be used for sleep maintenance with a sustained-release 1-mg preparation
- Hot bath or hot tub
- Breathing exercises and/or meditation to relax muscles and relieve tension

Most important, don't worry about lost sleep, since in most cases anxiety is what caused the problem in the first place. If you can learn to relax without drugs, you will have cured your sleeping problems while giving your immune system a powerful boost. Nearly all of the recommendations in chapters 5 and 6 will help you to achieve this goal.

One other important factor affecting sleep in a backache sufferer is a *comfortable mattress.* A mattress that is too soft and provides little support can add stress to the spine and back muscles. Although there is no scientific consensus on the best mattress for this condition, a recent survey of 238 orthopedic surgeons indicated that most (68 percent) would recommend a *firm* mattress for their patients with low back pain. According to the Better Sleep Council (a manufacturer's group), a mattress is "good" if it supports the natural curves of the body, particularly the spine and knees. This helps to maintain good sleeping posture. By contrast, poor sleeping positions can strain muscles and ligaments and increase the risk of compressed nerves and back pain. The American Chiropractic Association recommends using a mattress that has innerspring coils, which move independently to adjust to body curves, thereby keeping the spine in its natural position. The consensus seems to be that a good mattress for someone with backache (and for preventing it) is one that is comfortable (be sure to test it), firmer, supports your low back, and, to some degree, conforms to your body.

Relaxation is another essential ability that promotes physical health. Derived from the Latin *relaxare,* meaning "to loosen," relaxation is a way to allow the mind to return to a natural state of equilibrium, creating a state of balance between the right and left brain. It is also a highly effective means of stress reduction. Relaxation is a skill that can be improved upon with practice; therefore, it is recommended that you take time each day to relax. This can be achieved as easily as taking a few deep abdominal breaths or simply shifting your focus away from your problems and concerns, or through any activity that engages your creative and physical faculties. Such activities include reading and writing, gardening, taking a walk, painting, singing, playing music, doing crafts, or any other hobby that you enjoy for its own sake, without the need to be concerned about your performance. Committing two to three evening hours a week to the hobby or activity of your choice will help make relaxation a natural and regular part of your daily experience. The ability to relax and shift gears away from the competitive drive that compels most of us in our society holds the key to greater health

PROFESSIONAL CARE THERAPIES

Backache Survival is a book and a holistic treatment program with a self-care orientation. Whether or not you have made good progress on your own, you may still choose to avail yourself of several highly effective therapies for backache administered by a holistic physician or health care practitioner. From the survey on page 132, you learned that, to varying degrees, yoga, physical therapy, acupuncture, chiropractic, and osteopathic manipulation can be quite valuable in treating back pain. Since that survey was taken in 1985, I have personally practiced and experienced another highly effective modality—Healing Touch. The discipline of holistic medicine facilitates self-care while also including the prudent use of both conventional medicine and professional care alternatives. In addition to yoga, the following modalities are all potentially effective in long-term relief of backache.

Healing Touch

Healing Touch (HT) is a holistic therapy utilizing a variety of hands-on techniques to balance and realign the energy field within and surrounding the body. As HT clears and restores harmony to the energy system, it facilitates self-healing, affecting physical, emotional, and spiritual health. HT is used extensively in all areas of the nursing profession, from medical/surgical care, psychiatric, public health, hospice, pediatrics, to geriatric care.

The Healing Touch Program was developed by Janet Mentgen, R.N., B.S.N., who has been practicing energy-based care since 1980 in Denver, Colorado. HT was first offered as a pilot project at the University of Tennessee and in Gainesville, Florida, in 1989. It became a certificate program of the American Holistic Nurses Association in 1990; certification of HT practitioners and instructors began in 1993. Today, it is an international certification program (beginning to advanced levels) and continuing medical education program for nurses and massage therapists. In addition, physicians (myself included), social workers, counselors, body workers, and other health care practitioners are becoming trained and certified in this remarkably powerful therapeutic modality. There are currently nearly fifty studies, both completed and in progress, documenting its effectiveness. While some people prefer using HT for relief of acute symptoms, many work with the practitioner over several sessions to heal and deepen their understanding of chronic pain and/or illness. HT utilizes some of the techniques of Therapeutic Touch, along with the work of Brugh Joy, M.D., Barbara Brennan, Rosalyn Bruyere, and others. It is one of a few hands-on energy medicine modalities that also includes Reiki. Each of these therapies by itself can be helpful in treating backache.

In late 1986, I discovered that I had an exceptional ability to do Healing Touch and early the following year began using it with patients. When I started out with this new and obviously unconventional therapy, the first people I treated were friends and relatives. Among them was an athletic 33-year-old man with nearly incapacitating back pain, the result of an injury he sustained while doing construction work. He had pain radiating down one leg, with muscle weakness and loss of the knee reflex in that leg. He was diagnosed by his neurosurgeon as having a ruptured disc in his lumbar spine and was scheduled to have surgery two weeks following his HT treatment. I did a 15- to 20-minute HT treatment on his low back on three consecutive days. Each day his pain was substantially diminished, and by the time he left on the third day it was almost completely gone. Several days later he returned to his physician for a presurgical visit, and the neurosurgeon was surprised and perplexed by what he saw. His examination revealed a normal reflex and improved muscle strength, along with the continued absence of pain. He canceled the surgery, and my friend has remained free of back pain ever since. He's continued to do some back stretching exercises, but at age 49 he remains quite active. He still skis regularly, rows rafts on the Colorado River, and plays basketball. This experience was one of several similarly remarkable healing successes using HT that inspired me to deepen my commitment to the practice of holistic medicine, and especially to the holistic health modality of Healing Touch.

Trigger Point Injection Therapy (TPIT) and Myotherapy

This is a highly effective treatment for backache developed by Janet Travell, M.D., during the 1940s. During the Kennedy and Johnson administrations, she became the first female physician to serve at the White House, and was instrumental in enabling President Kennedy to cope with back injuries sustained during World War II. Her work is based on "trigger points," chronically sore or irritated areas in the muscles caused by physical trauma, stress, disease, structural imbalances, or chronic overuse. In response to such stresses, muscles contract and, over time, settle into a holding pattern that can trigger chronic pain. Through the injection of saline or procaine (anesthetic) solutions, Travell's TPIT technique is able to release these patterns of contraction, resulting in elimination or reduction of pain.

Similar results can be obtained by applying deep pressure to the trigger points without the injections. This technique was developed by Bonnie Prudden in the mid-1970s. She was one of the original members of the President's Council on Physical Fitness and Sports in the 1950s, and her work has become known as Prudden Myotherapy. This hands-on therapy relieves muscle pain quickly and cost effectively and can be taught to patients to apply to themselves. The self-care aspect of this technique allows it to be effective for long-term relief of backache.

Prolotherapy

Also known as *regenerative therapy* or *sclerotherapy*, prolotherapy is a technique that can significantly reduce or eliminate back pain. The technique involves the injection of a substance such as dextrose (a small quantity of diluted sugar water) with a local anesthetic such as lidocaine into the area of pain in order to stimulate the body's natural healing processes via the production of collagen, which strengthens the weakened area and reduces pain. One to four prolotherapy treatments administered by a skilled practitioner are often enough to relieve pain. This therapy is applicable to all musculoskeletal pain problems, including arthritis and headaches. There are several studies documenting its effectiveness.

Osteopathic Medicine

As an osteopathic physician, I'm most familiar with the art and science of healing of osteopathic medicine, which is essentially the same as *holistic* medicine. It was founded and developed by Andrew Taylor Still, M.D., in 1874. The D.O. degree stands for Doctor of Osteopathic Medicine, and D.O.s are fully licensed physicians with unlimited rights and privileges to practice in all fifty states in the United States. D.O.s who have graduated from an osteopathic medical school have completed at a minimum a four-year undergraduate degree, four years of osteopathic medical education at one of the nineteen accredited osteopathic medical schools, and usually several years of residency training, depending upon their specialty and area of expertise. D.O.s practice in all medical and surgical specialties, with the greatest percentage of practitioners being in primary care—family practice, pediatrics, and internal medicine.

A. T. Still was a fourth-generation M.D. who, after losing his wife and three of his own children one winter to an epidemic of meningitis, began to question the completeness of his medical training. He also suffered from terrible headaches, for which he had found no solution in the medical model of his day. In the truly Hippocratic tradition, he became a seeker of answers to his own challenging medical problem. He became widely known for his effective, noninvasive, hands-on approach and was referred to as a "bone-setter." Dr. Still's intention was simply to improve quality and raise the standard of care, not to create a new school of medicine. However, he was unsuccessful in his attempts to have his ideas and methods incorporated into the traditional medical model. Since his apprentices (seven-year apprenticeships were the accepted method of medical training in his day) were being taught medical "heresy," they were not granted the traditional M.D. degree. Instead, they were called D.O.s—Doctors of Osteopathy. (The Latin root *osteo* means "bone," and *patheia* is Greek for "passion" or "suffering.")

When medical schools opened around the turn of the twentieth century, osteopathic students were still thought to be medical heretics, and thus began the two different forms of complete medical training with two separate medical degrees—M.D. and D.O. Today, osteopathic medical schools have a very similar four-year curriculum to allopathic schools, with most of the same courses and textbooks but with several profound differences. Osteopathic medicine has, at its core, a holistic philosophy and a highly developed system of manual diagnostics and treatment techniques that are designed to stimulate our own innate healing and homeostatic mechanisms. The holistic principles upon which osteopathic medicine was founded are as follows:

(1) *A person is a complete dynamic unit of function, comprising body, mind, and spirit.* Osteopathic medicine recognizes the im-

portance and uniqueness of each of these three elements in every individual and their relationship to disease and optimal health.

(2) *The body possesses self-regulatory mechanisms that are self-healing in nature.* The primary objective of the osteopathic physician is to remove the obstacles to health, thereby enabling the body to seek its own path back toward health.

(3) *Structure and function are interrelated at all levels.* Therefore, if there is an asymmetry, restriction of motion, or tissue texture change present (these are called "somatic dysfunctions" by osteopathic physicians), one can predict a subsequent alteration in function of the same or referred regions.

(4) *Rational treatment is based on understanding and integrating the previous three principles.* Osteopathic medicine, in fact, offers a unique way of looking at patients and their disease. It is based upon a *whole person* perspective, an awareness that the body can heal itself and that its natural state is one of *optimal health,* combined with a scientific focus on understanding and treating the *causes* of disease.

Osteopathic manipulative treatment, or OMT, is as much an art as it is a science, and therefore each patient with backache may be treated a bit differently by an osteopathic physician. A thorough osteopathic structural exam from foot to head should precede any assumptions that all cases of low back pain have their origins in the lumbar spine. This means that, because of the interconnectedness of the body, the painful back could possibly manifest symptoms as a result of compensating for a primary structural problem elsewhere in the body, which might be obstructing the flow of blood and nutrients into the low back. If other primary problem sites are not ruled out and/or diagnosed and treated appropriately, the low back could be treated repeatedly without significant improvement. This is often the case when one forgets that the body is a complete unit. Attempting to segment it often results in inadequate or unsuccessful treatment.

Osteopathic manipulative treatment is often highly effective for backache from a variety of causes, but especially those related to mechanical and/or postural origin. OMT helps patients relieve the underlying imbalances causing these problems by diagnosing and treating the observable or palpable physical changes (the somatic dysfunctions) that are present. When a somatic dysfunction is successfully treated with OMT, there is usually a significant decrease in the intensity, duration, and frequency of pain. Other positive outcomes associated with OMT treatment include a lessening of muscle tension along with better spinal balance, improved local as well as overall flexibility, and normalized circulation. Several studies on patients with both acute and chronic low back pain have shown OMT to be more effective than standard medical treatment—that is, medication. There is also an added benefit of a diminished requirement for drugs to relieve pain, along with their potentially unpleasant side effects.

There are many types of osteopathic manipulative techniques that are used to treat back pain. The most effective and commonly used for backache are the following:

- Counterstrain
- Facilitated positional release
- Ligamentous articular release
- Cranial osteopathy—Also known as *osteopathy in the cranial field* or *craniosacral therapy,* this is a system of diagnosis and treatment originally described and developed by William Garner Sutherland, D.O. He graduated from the American School of Osteopathy in 1900 and worked on developing what would become cranial osteopathy over the next fifty-plus years. His first publication on this subject was called *The Cranial Bowl* and was published in 1939. The underlying principles behind cranial osteopathy are the following:

- There is an inherent motion of the brain and spinal cord.
- There is regular fluctuation of the cerebrospinal fluid.
- There is inherent mobility of the intracranial and intraspinal membranes.
- There is articular mobility of the cranial bones.

- There is involuntary mobility of the sacrum between the hip bones.

A practitioner of cranial osteopathy evaluates and treats the entire body of the patient but is particularly good at diagnosing and addressing structural alterations in the head and sacrum (the bone at the base of the spine). This approach can be of significant benefit to a person who has acute back pain due to a structural or neurophysiologic problem, since the cranial technique is very gentle and rarely induces pain. It usually works well in cases of low back pain, since there are always areas of sacral and lumbar dysfunction, and this technique is excellent for treating these.

One of my osteopathic colleagues, Todd Bezilla, D.O., is a former member of the faculty at the Philadelphia College of Osteopathic Medicine and taught in the department of osteopathic manual medicine (OMM). He has been a valuable contributor to several of my books, including this section of *Backache Survival*. He has successfully treated numerous patients with backache using OMT, including several who avoided surgery with diagnosed herniated discs. The following is the story of one of his patients, as described by Dr. Bezilla.

John was a 56-year-old man who came to see me on referral for constant pain in his low back, hips, and legs, along with a diagnosis of severe osteoarthritis, degenerative disc disease, and spinal stenosis of his lumbar spine. He worked as a truck driver doing deliveries, which also required him to intermittently lift and carry materials that weighed up to 75 pounds. He had been placed on a variety of medications including NSAIDs and non-narcotic analgesics, as well as Neurontin, in the months prior to his first office visit. He was very concerned that he would not be able to continue his job, earn money, and provide for himself and his wife. He noted that he didn't want to have surgery if he didn't have to, although the constant pain was starting to make him think that it wouldn't be such a bad idea. I evaluated and treated him using very gentle techniques including craniosacral. I taught his wife how to perform a lumbosacral release and encouraged her to perform it daily with him at home. I had him restrict his driving and lifting, gave him specific spinal mobility exercises to perform at home, and had him return in two weeks. He returned with his wife excited to report that, to his amazement, this treatment was working. I reevaluated him and treated him with more OMT. He was able to tolerate slightly more vigorous treatment this time, and I was successful at freeing some motion using LVHA (low velocity, high amplitude) and myofascial release techniques. I encouraged him to maintain his home program and stressed the importance of his wife continuing to administer the treatments that I had taught her. She was very happy to continue and stated she was amazed at the changes in his back that she was able to feel with her hands. I told her that perhaps she had missed her calling. We laughed and they left. They returned once more a few weeks later and noted that he had been able to discontinue most of his pain medicines and was back to full-duty at work. Unfortunately, however, his wife had fallen and broken her treating arm, but was still treating him with her other hand. I told him that as long as he was doing well and his wife was able to continue the back treatments, he should come back only as needed. I haven't had to treat him since.

The treatment of this patient with backache, osteoarthritis, degenerative disc disease, and spinal stenosis serves as an excellent example of the therapeutic value of osteopathic manipulative therapy. Although he was free of back pain, had eliminated all medication, and was able to return to his strenuous job, he probably did not grossly change any of the underlying degenerative pathology causing his chronic problem. And even though he did not commit to a major life overhaul, he did to some extent experience holistic medical treatment. His belief about overcoming the problem changed dramatically with the first sign of significant improvement. His subsequent optimism helped speed his recovery. The fact that his wife was an integral part of his treatment I'm sure must have strengthened their marital bond and allowed her to feel good about her valuable contribution to his recovery. The healing effect of love is the foundation of the practice of holistic medicine, and touch is probably the most direct and powerful means of conveying love. In spite of the fact that OMT is technically a professional care therapy, in this instance it was administered by a nonprofessional (who was taught by a D.O.) and worked quite well.

This story illustrates the type of patient who, when confronted with a painful recurrence of his backache, is often receptive to going further with the holistic treatment program. A quick fix for a chronic problem that results from a degenerative process, such as arthritis, usually offers only temporary relief. But when chronic back pain is the result of a structural or mechanical problem, OMT is nearly always successful in allowing for greater overall function and a long-term reduction in pain. Regardless of the therapy, if it's not used in conjunction with a holistic—body, mind, spirit—approach, it will not address the multiple causes nor will it be as effective in producing long-lasting improvement of backache. It is also true that many people with chronic low back pain will gradually see a resolution of their pain without doing anything. This can occur as a result of the body's adaptation to the structural changes. However, that individual is typically more susceptible to further injury and pain in the future. OMT, along with yoga, stretching, strengthening, and other therapies, can help allow the body to adapt in the best manner possible. In many cases, the backache sufferer will have a much healthier back than before the onset of the back pain.

To find an osteopathic physician in your area, contact the American Academy of Osteopathy at (317) 879-1881.

Chiropractic

Developed over one hundred years ago by David Daniel Palmer, chiropractic (Greek for "done by hand") has as its goal the maintenance of the health of the nervous system through the adjustment of bones and joints. Chiropractic theory holds that spinal misalignment (called "subluxation") interferes with the flow of vital energy or, what Palmer described as the body's "innate intelligence." Since the nervous system's primary pathway is along the spine, when any part of the spine is subluxated, nerve impulses can be impeded and eventually result in dis-ease in the body's various organs. Chiropractors (or D.C.s) restore spinal alignment with a variety of adjustment and manipulation techniques and compose a large portion of the alternative practitioners in the United States. Patients with backache spend more on chiropractic care than for any other alternative therapy. Many chiropractors also use kinesiology (muscle testing) and provide nutritional counseling in their practices.

Chiropractic can be very helpful in treating both acute and chronic low back pain. Chiropractic manipulation helps to self-correct abnormal ranges of motion in the spine and extremities. Most low back pain either directly or indirectly involves the motion of the vertebral unit, which comprises two vertebrae and its associated joints, discs, and ligaments. A chiropractor will first attempt to identify the cause of your back pain and to treat you as a whole person. The treatment of nearly all cases of low back pain involves taking a history, a careful physical exam, including a postural examination, followed by proper testing. Most chiropractors believe that poor posture is a primary cause of low back pain. This results in gross muscle imbalance in the trunk and lower extremities, causing abnormal biomechanics and stress to the low back. A chiropractic examination of a patient with chronic low back pain often presents with the following muscular findings: weak lower abdominals, short or long hamstrings and/or hip flexors and hip rotators, and weak dynamic stabilizers of the lower leg and foot.

A chiropractor may offer recommended exercises, ergonomic suggestions, and nutritional advice, in addition to comprehensive treatment that may, or may not, include manipulation. If you're considering chiropractic treatment but are unsure, I would recommend that you have a chiropractor assess your posture and suggest exercises to you. This is usually not expensive, and this one visit may be all you'll need to get started on a simple exercise and strengthening program to help you correct your posture and relieve your pain.

To find a chiropractor in your area, contact the American Chiropractic Association at (800) 986-4636.

Traditional Chinese Medicine

Traditional Chinese medicine is the primary health care system currently used by approximately 30 percent of the world's population. It is believed to be one of the oldest medical systems in existence, dating back almost 5,000 years. The practice of acupuncture (a method of using fine needles to stimulate invisible lines of energy running beneath the surface of the skin) is the component of Chinese medicine most familiar to Americans, but the system also includes Chinese herbology, moxabustion (the burning of an herb at acupuncture points), massage, diet, exercise, and meditation.

In ancient China, doctors were not paid if patients under their care became sick. The job of the physician was to keep patients healthy. Chinese medicine believes that a certain process happens before the body develops a problem or disease. A Chinese medicine practitioner (O.M.D., Doctor of Oriental Medicine) looks for this process or pattern of disharmony. Through questioning, observation, and palpation, a practitioner can determine a person's current state of health and the problems that that individual will be at highest risk for developing in the future. In this way, Chinese medicine is an effective preventive therapy.

Traditional Chinese medicine is based on a history, philosophy, and sociology very different from that of the West. Over thousands of years, it has developed a unique understanding of how the body works. Practitioners of Chinese medicine see disease as an imbalance between the body's nutritive substances, called "yin," and the functional activity of the body, called "yang." This imbalance causes a disruption of the flow of vital energy that circulates through pathways in the body known as "meridians." This vital energy, called *qi* ("chi,") keeps the blood circulating, warms the body, and fights disease. The intimate connection between the organ systems of the body and the meridians enables the practice of acupuncture to intercede and rebalance the body's energy through stimulation of specific points along the meridians.

People who have used Chinese medicine for a particular physical symptom frequently experience improvement in seemingly unrelated problems. This occurs because the Chinese approach tends to restore the body to a greater degree of balance, thereby enhancing its capacity for self-healing. The entire person is treated, not just the symptom; the relationship of body, mind, emotions, spirit, and environment are all taken into account.

The World Health Organization has published a list of over fifty diseases successfully treated with acupuncture. Included on the list are low back pain, sciatica, arthritis, sinusitis, asthma, the common cold, headaches (including migraine), constipation, and diarrhea. Acupuncture has also been effective in the treatment of allergies, addictions, insomnia, stress, depression, infertility, and menstrual problems.

Chinese herbs are the most common element of Chinese medicine as it is currently practiced in China. The herbs are becoming more popular in the United States, but it is still much easier to find a licensed acupuncturist (L.Ac., C.A., R.Ac., Dipl. Ac.) than an O.M.D. who is knowledgeable about Chinese herbs as well as acupuncture. Since 1995, there has been national board certification in Chinese herbal medicine, offering the degree Dipl. C.H. As more schools of traditional Chinese medicine are established in this country, these licensed practitioners will be much easier to find.

Pharmaceutical drugs are usually made by synthetically producing the active ingredient of an herb. Medicinal plants differ from the isolated active ingredients in synthetic drugs because they contain associate substances that balance the medicinal effects. Uncomfortable side effects are generally the result of the removal of these associate substances. Chinese herbs are capable of regenerating, vitalizing, and balancing the vital energy, tissue, and organs of the body without harmful side effects. They can be taken in pill or powder form or as raw herbs made into tea.

In traditional Chinese medicine, emphasis is placed on ensuring that a person's energy and blood flow are smooth and harmonious. In people with backache, the flow of blood and energy (*qi*) has been disrupted, which can cause pain. Additionally, in accordance with Chinese medicine theory, the kidney system (channel/meridian) "governs" the low back. The urinary bladder meridian also affects the low back. In conditions that affect the spine and bones, specifically their formation and integrity, there is a weakness in the kidney system.

There are two primary types of people with kidney weaknesses. The more common type are those who are yin deficient. They are "hot" and might complain of night sweats or tend to sweat excessively. The most common characteristics of the *warm kidney yin-deficient* person are the following: they like caffeine, alcohol, stimulants, or amphetamines; they exercise a lot, have heightened sexual energy, take ibuprofen, and enjoy saunas and hot tubs (sweating). All of these things will continue to weaken the kidney, so it is recommended that they be avoided or minimized. The *cold kidney yang-deficient* individual might manifest symptoms of being cold, fatigue, nighttime urination, impotence, and low blood pressure. These people should avoid Nutrasweet, cold liquids and cold food, coffee and caffeine, and stimulants and amphetamines. They are also told to keep the kidney area of their low back warm.

There can be many associated factors affecting the development and progression of backache. When seeking treatment from an acupuncturist/Chinese medicine doctor, these factors will be taken into consideration. The primary focus of treatment is to move and regulate the flow of energy (*qi*) and blood, and support the kidney energy. The acupuncture treatment itself is relatively painless. Five to fifteen needles are placed along the appropriate meridians that stimulate the release of endorphins (the body's natural painkiller) and allow for the free flow of *qi*.

One excellent study documenting the beneficial effects of acupuncture followed fifty patients with chronic low back pain. They were divided into two groups—one received acupuncture right away, and the other was scheduled to receive it later. Of the immediately treated group, 83 percent improved, reducing their average pain scores by half. In the delayed treatment group, before treatment began, one third improved and one quarter got worse. After receiving acupuncture, 75 percent of this group also improved. Forty weeks later, 58 percent of the patients who had received acupuncture (in either group) continued to show improvement. In 1997, the National Institutes of Health (NIH) issued a report acknowledging that acupuncture can be helpful in treating low back pain.

Simple self-care treatments for backache are available by using a few topical products that usually can be purchased at a health food store. They include Zheng Gu Shul (a linament that should only be used by the warm kidney yin-deficient group), an antilumbago tablet, and Chinese herbal plasters.

To find an acupuncturist in your area, contact the National Commission for the Certification of Acupuncturists at (202) 232-1404.

Bodywork and Body Movement

The various therapies within the category of bodywork and body movement all focus on restoring structural alignment and posture, creating unrestricted movement, and relieving physical tension and stress. As a result, each one of them, depending upon the individual, can be helpful in treating backache.

Therapeutic massage is perhaps the most researched form of bodywork, offering a wide range of scientifically supported benefits. One study in 2001 compared acupuncture, therapeutic massage, and self-care education for chronic low back pain. The participants in the study received therapeutic massage for ten weeks and experienced greater symptom relief than those who received acupuncture treatments or self-care educational materials.

Massage also appears to be highly effective for temporary relief (see page 132). Massage was an integral part of many ancient cultures, including China, India, Persia, Arabia, and Greece. There are an estimated eighty forms of massage therapy available in the United States today, with only about twenty that are more than twenty years old. The best known is European massage, of which Swedish is the most popular. It involves long gliding strokes, kneading, and friction. It helps back pain by relaxing tense, painful muscles; improving circulation; raising levels of endorphins, the body's natural pain-killing compounds; promoting general relaxation; and restoring flexibility and range of motion. This type of massage typically works on the body's superficial layers of musculature. Massage from a spouse or partner can be helpful, but it's better to find a therapist who has received formal training and who is either nationally certified or is affiliated with a national organization that promotes professional standards. To find a massage therapist in your area, contact the American Massage Therapy Association at (847) 864-0123.

Rolfing, more properly known as Structural Integration, is the best known of the deep-tissue techniques of bodywork. It was developed by Ida Rolf, Ph.D. (1896–1979). Her doctorate in biochemistry and physiology, combined with years of study of other bodywork techniques, led her to conclude that all physiological function is an expression of structure. Her belief led her to develop her own system of bodywork as a way to cure her spinal arthritis. She realized that the physiologic conditions that contributed to causing arthritis could be resolved by stretching fascial tissues.

In Rolf's view, a body that is poorly aligned must struggle to maintain balance in the face of gravitational pull. As it does so, the body tends to compensate for areas of imbalance or misalignment in one area through adaptive changes in other areas. Over time, according to Rolfers (as practitioners of Rolfing are called), such compensation leads to an overall weakening of the body's entire structure, resulting in compromised body function. The aim of Rolfing is to restore the body to proper alignment so that all of its sections—head, neck, shoulders, torso, hips, legs, ankles, and feet—correspond and interact correctly with gravity. Rolf maintained that when the body's alignment was restored, all systems of the body are able to operate more efficiently, thereby improving total well-being.

Depending upon the degree of misalignment, Rolfing can take several months or even years to fully restore optimal positioning and function. During a Rolfing session, deep pressure is applied to the *fascia,* layers of connective tissue that hold and support the body's muscles and bones and cover muscle fibers and internal organs. Due to injury and chronic stress, the fascia can shorten or become overly thick as a result of the body's adaptive coping strategies. Poor posture, disease, and emotional trauma can also contort the fascia. As a consequence, rigidity or oversolidity can occur, leading to habitual body distortion, spinal misalignment, limited range of motion, and repressed emotions. Rolfers seek to reestablish proper alignment and improved mobility by loosening and manipulating the fascia, using their fingers, thumbs, and sometimes elbows.

Rolfing, like most forms of bodywork, does not focus on treating specific symptoms. Rather, emphasis is placed on bringing the body back into alignment with gravity by restoring the fascia to its natural state of elasticity. Although Rolfers make no claims of being able to treat specific disease conditions, Rolfing has been quite helpful in alleviating conditions of chronic pain and muscular tension, including low back pain, and in improving posture. I've personally experienced dramatic (although temporary) relief of back pain of ten days' duration following a Rolfing session. After curing her arthritis, Ida Rolf commented that "many diagnoses of 'arthritis' reflect nothing more serious than a shortened or displaced muscle or ligament resulting from a recent or not-so-recent traumatic episode." I have had many Rolfing sessions with Jaison Kayn, a student of Ida Rolf, and found them to be one of the most powerful holistic therapies (that is, benefiting body, mind, and spirit) I've ever experienced. To find a Rolfer in your area, contact the International Rolf Institute at (303) 449-5903.

Caution: Due to its deep manipulation of tissues, Rolfing is not advised for anyone suffering from acute pain or diseases due to underlying bone weakness, such as osteoporosis or fracture. Patients suffering from organic or inflammatory conditions, such as cancer or rheumatoid arthritis, or from acute skin inflammation, should also forgo Rolfing treatment.

Hellerwork, another deep-tissue technique, was developed by Joseph Heller, one of Ida Rolf's early students and the first president of the Rolf Institute. Besides employing deep-touch techniques similar to those used by Rolfers to structurally realign the body, Hellerwork practitioners also seek to impart to their clients a greater awareness of the relationship between mind and body. To this end, they utilize movement reeducation techniques and verbal dialogue to address the complex interrelationship between the body's mechanical, psychological, and energetic functioning.

Hellerwork usually consists of eleven sessions, each of which lasts for 90 minutes and makes use of a thematic approach that is geared toward providing clients with a structure for organizing the emotional aspects of the work. In the first session, for example, treatment is focused on resolving tension and unconscious holding patterns in the chest in order to bring about fuller, more natural breathing. During this session, a Hellerwork practitioner will typically also engage clients in a dialogue meant to call attention to his or her attitudes and emotions that might be affecting the breathing process. Instruction in proper movement is also provided in order to train the client in more efficient ways of using the body's energy and minimizing mechanical stress. Clients learn how to stand, sit, walk, run, and lift objects in a manner that is best suited to their own physiology. Videotaping a client's movements might also be used to provide feedback and a clearer understanding of how movement patterns may need to be corrected. This form of bodywork can also be very helpful in treating backache. To find a Hellerwork practitioner in your area, contact the Associated Bodywork and Massage Professionals at (800) 458-2267.

The *Feldenkrais Method* was developed by physicist and engineer Moshe Feldenkrais after he suffered a serious knee injury. Rather than undergo surgery, Feldenkrais devoted himself to the study of the nervous system and human behavior. His research, along with his knowledge of physiology, anatomy, psychology, neurology, and the martial arts, led him to conclude that a person's self-image is crucial to how he or she thinks and functions in the world. In Feldenkrais's view, the human organism is a complex, interrelated system of function and intelligence in which all movement reflects the condition of the nervous system as well as being the basis of self-awareness.

Central to the philosophy of the Feldenkrais Method is the belief that the central nervous system can be retrained, resulting in improved patterns of behavior and movement. Feldenkrais also emphasized the importance of proper breathing, viewing the breath as an essential aspect of movement. In order to help his students overcome a lifetime of habitual limiting movement and breathing patterns, Feldenkrais developed two teaching methods: Functional Integration and Awareness through Movement.

Functional Integration is taught individually in hour-long sessions tailored to the specific needs of each client. Using gentle manipulation and movement exercises, practitioners guide clients through new, easier, and more efficient ways of moving. No attempt is made to alter the client's body structure. Instead, practitioners use touch to help clients discover their own most appropriate movement style.

Awareness through Movement classes are taught in a group setting. Classes average 45 to 60 minutes, during which time students are guided through a series of directed movements. By paying attention to each exercise, students acquire a greater awareness of how they move and of any unnecessary tension their movements may have. The exercises are gentle and often subtle, such as lifting one foot slightly off the floor. They may be performed while sitting or lying on the floor, standing, or while seated, and can be accompanied by verbal cues or imagery designed to facilitate a deeper awareness of how each student moves. All exercises are performed slowly, without straining.

Using the Feldenkrais Method to confront low back pain offers an opportunity to explore a path of somatic learning not typical of our societal orientation toward "exercise." In our predominantly "no pain, no gain" fitness orientation, strength and stretching are the usual vehicles for improvement. The Feldenkrais somatic learning approach relies upon ease, comfort, flow, and gentleness as the primary sensate signals for improvement.

These signals are evoked through small, gentle oscillations rather than stretching or holding positions.

These Feldenkrais oscillations reflect early childhood patterns of somatic learning through movement that are the foundation of all future development. Our cultural bias is to pay attention to the outer form of the "exercise" through concentration and a type of tunnel vision. Feldenkrais gently compels an effortless, inner attention that is mobile and nonexclusive. Hence, the pelvic tilt becomes a pelvic tilting—that is, a dynamic, small, gentle series of oscillations that requires a sort of split-screen lensing for skeletal ease and release of extra-muscular tensions. In print this may sound complex, but in practice it is easy, imaginative, comfortable, and effective.

Essential to the effectiveness of the Feldenkrais Method is cultivating a willingness to "listen" to the somatic feedback ever present in our bodies but rarely heeded; for example, if it hurts, do less: gentler, smaller, slower. This awareness response is counterintuitive to our cultural learning around physical education, that bigger is better, with the "no pain, no gain" approach. A greater capacity for movements to become large, fast, and powerful can emerge from the Feldenkrais somatic explorations, but only after the chronic/acute condition abates. A low back crisis can often be a remarkable opportunity not only to learn a new approach to working with physical challenges but also, through the conscious, methodical alleviation of suffering, to come to know oneself better. I have personally experienced the therapeutic benefit of Feldenkrais in treating back pain through my work with Lawrence Phillips, a gifted teacher and healer. To find a Feldenkrais practitioner in your area, contact the Feldenkrais Guild of North America at (800) 755-2118.

The *Trager Approach,* or Trager Work, was developed by U.S. physician Milton Trager, M.D., a specialist in neuromuscular conditions and a former boxer, acrobat, and dancer. Trager theorized that pain and other health conditions could be permanently resolved by bypassing the conscious mind to access the unconscious mind directly. Although different from the Feldenkrais Method, the goals of the Trager Approach are largely the same: releasing chronic and habitual tension in the body by helping clients recognize and interrupt limiting or inefficient movement patterns and correcting poor posture. One result of the attainment of these goals is less restricted movement and blood flow to a painful low back.

The Trager Approach is distinguished by the playful quality of its work, which achieves its goals through gentle, rhythmic touch and movement exercises. As the work is performed, the client lies passively on a massage table or flat surface, letting the practitioner guide the movements from a meditative state known as "hook up," which enables him or her to more deeply perceive the client's flow of energy. Limbs are lightly cradled and moved about in order to retrain the unconscious, via the nervous system, to move beyond old patterns of restriction and holding into a state of greater flexibility and ease. To find a Trager Approach practitioner in your area, contact The Trager Institute at (216) 896-9383.

Note: The Trager Approach is safe for most people but should be avoided in cases of broken bones, fever, blood clotting, problem pregnancies, and certain forms of cancer where manipulation might contribute to the spread of the disease.

The *Pilates Method* is currently one of the most popular therapies for chronic low back pain. It was developed in the early 1900s by a German-born athlete and physical therapist, Joseph Hubertus Pilates, after years of practicing yoga, meditation, and the physical fitness practices of the ancient Greeks. After experimenting with physical therapy techniques, he developed the specialized equipment that provides the foundation of his Pilates program. Shortly after he emigrated to the United States, his work soon attracted injured ballet dancers in the New York City Ballet. It is designed to repattern range of motion, realign poor posture, rehabilitate injuries, heal chronic back and neck pain, diminish stress, and prevent injury. Because of its mind–body focus, some people have described it as "a Western yoga with equipment." A precise set of movements is coordinated with breathing and eventually can become both graceful and aerobic. A primary objective of Pilates is to teach people to use their body correctly while improving posture, increasing body strength, flexibility, and coordination. It targets the muscles close to the body's core—the lower, deep abdominals and back muscles—to create a firm foundation for movement.

Other Complementary Therapies

Homeopathic remedies that have proven to be helpful in treating acute low back pain include arnica as a topical cream or taken orally (especially effective for sprains and strains), Rhus tox, and Ruta graveolens. Aconite can be taken when the pain comes on suddenly or in cold or dry weather.

Magnets have in recent years become popular for backache, but to my knowledge there are no studies documenting their effectiveness. However, they are safe to use and are usually worn in belts or taped across the back. They can also be placed in mattresses. There is no harm in trying them, and I've heard from a number of people that they've been quite helpful in relieving back pain.

SUMMARY

The entire physical health component of the Backache Survival Program is too comprehensive for anyone to be expected to immediately follow every one of these recommendations. However, there are many people who have obtained significant relief from their backache by initially strictly adhering to just one of the components of the program—particularly yoga. My suggestion to patients is to make a *commitment* to incorporate into your daily life as many of the above recommendations as you are comfortably able to do. Take your time. The more gradual the process, the more likely it is that you'll stay with it. Try adding one new thing each week.

If you have followed the Backache Survival Program closely

for at least two months, you will most likely have noticed a significant improvement in the condition of your back. If so, you can begin gradually to increase your level of exercise. Every individual is somewhat different, and you'll have to find the appropriate level for you. If your back pain begins to recur, then decrease to your previous exercise regime.

If, after two months of consistently adhering (daily practice) to at least three of the recommendations in this chapter, you have not yet experienced any change in your symptoms, I suggest that you consider one of the professional care therapies or consult with a holistic physician.

Committing yourself to a consistent program of breathing and eating well, taking the proper supplements, drinking enough water, and becoming more physically fit based on the recommendations in this chapter will enable you to achieve improvements in your physical well-being and with your backache in as little as a few weeks. You will have relaxed the muscles and relieved inflammation while enhancing blood flow and strengthening the tissues of your low back. And you will have addressed some of the causes of your back pain. Before long, you will find that your reserves of energy are greater and that you are physically stronger, more powerful, and more flexible. You will also develop a more positive self-image and feel better about how your body looks and performs in every realm of activity. And if you have been spending more time outdoors, you will feel more connected to and empowered by nature.

Optimal physical health is a feeling of *harmony* within your body. The underlying physical basis will be experienced as an *effortless flowing of all bodily functions and fluids.* Your breathing will become more abdominal and less restricted, providing a greater supply of oxygen to every cell as it flows through less constricted arteries. Enhanced by an increased intake of water, your circulation will in turn allow your kidneys and bowels more complete elimination of toxins and waste. Your nutritious diet will provide better nourishment and more energy to your cells. And your more regular and effortless bowel movements will be more conducive to maximum absorption of nutrients. Your body movement, stretching, and exercise programs will even further facilitate the nourishment of all cells, tissues, and organs.

As you begin to thrive, you will be sleeping more deeply and making time for relaxation. You will enjoy greater sexual energy and often greater endurance and pleasure. You will become more aware and appreciative of the miracle of your own body and the intelligence and efficiency with which it regulates and heals itself. You will also have a better understanding of how your body relates to and is impacted by the environment surrounding it. You might even develop a sense of how the improved harmony with your environment may enhance your longevity.

Your body is simply working better. As a result, it can provide you with some of life's simplest but greatest pleasures: deep sleep, uncongested breathing, graceful movement without pain, unrestricted urination, easy bowel movements, sexual intercourse, and an awareness of the unimpeded flow of life energy that connects us to one another and to our environment. Such benefits are just the beginning of your journey to optimal well-being. They will continue to become more noticeable as you take more responsibility for your health and follow this chapter's guidelines in the months and years ahead. In the process, you will be creating the foundation necessary for healing the other aspects of holistic medicine's triumvirate—*mind* and *spirit*—while you are healing your aching back.

Chapter 5

HEALING YOUR MIND

The greatest discovery of any generation is that human beings can alter their lives by altering the attitudes of their minds.

ALBERT SCHWEITZER

COMPONENTS OF MENTAL HEALTH

Peace of mind and contentment

- A job that you love doing
- Optimism
- A sense of humor
- Financial well-being
- Living your life vision
- The ability to express your creativity and talents
- The capacity to make healthy decisions

COMPONENTS OF EMOTIONAL HEALTH

Self-acceptance and high self-esteem

- The capacity to identify, express, experience, and accept all of your feelings, both painful and joyful
- Awareness of the intimate connection between your physical and emotional bodies
- The ability to confront your greatest fears
- The fulfillment of your capacity to play
- Peak experiences on a regular basis

One of the most exciting developments in the field of medicine in recent decades has been the scientific verification that our physical health is directly influenced by our thoughts and emotions. The reverse is also true: Overwhelming evidence now exists showing that our physiology has a direct correlation to the ways we habitually think and feel. While Eastern systems of medicine, such as traditional Chinese medicine and Ayurveda, have for centuries recognized these facts and stressed the importance of a harmonious connection between body and mind, in the West this mind–body connection did not begin to be acknowledged until research conducted in the 1970s and '80s conclusively revealed the ability of thoughts, emotions, and attitudes to influence our bodies' immune functions. In fact, many of the scientists exploring this relatively new field of psychoneuroimmunology (PNI) have concluded that *there is no separation between mind and body.*

In order to heal our minds and emotions, it helps to know what we mean by the term "mental health." From the perspective of holistic medicine, the essence of mental health is peace of mind and feelings of contentment. Being mentally healthy means that you recognize the ways in which your thoughts, beliefs, mental imagery, and attitudes affect your well-being and limit or expand your ability to enjoy your life. It also means knowing that you always have choices about what you think and believe, being aware of your gifts, practicing your special talents, working at a job that you enjoy, and being clear about your priorities, values, and goals. People who have made a commitment to their mental health live their lives with rich reserves of humor and optimism. They have chosen a nurturing set of beliefs and attitudes that fill them with peace and hope. Most people who buy this book do so with the belief, however minimal, that they or a loved one will not have to suffer with backache for the rest of their lives and will free themselves of living with the fear of chronic and, at times, incapacitating pain. Since you have read to this point and begun practicing the physical components of the Backache Survival Program, your belief has probably been strengthened considerably. You can determine your own state of mental health by referring to the appropriate section of the Wellness Self-Test in Chapter 3, and then use the information in this chapter to improve the areas you may need to work on.

The term "mental health" can be interpreted to include not only our thoughts and beliefs but also our feelings. However, when your focus is specifically on "feelings," this is the realm of *emotional health.* These aspects of ourselves—*mental* and *emotional*—are for the most part inextricably related and together form the "mind" aspect of holistic health. As your healing journey progresses, you will increasingly come to recognize how your own distorted or illogical thoughts (often rooted in the past) are the underlying cause of feelings such as anger, depression, anxiety, fear, and unfounded guilt. Learning how to free yourself from such distorted thinking patterns is the goal of this chapter—and of behavioral medicine, the aspect of holistic medicine that deals with this interconnectedness between physical, mental, and emotional health. Behavioral medicine includes professional treatment approaches such as *psychotherapy, mind-body medicine, guided imagery and visualization, biofeedback therapy, hypnotherapy, neurolinguistic programming* (NLP), *Healing Touch and other energy therapies, orthomolecular medicine* (the use of nutritional supplements to treat chronic mental dis-ease), *flower essences,* and body-centered therapies like *Rolfing* and *Hellerwork.*

With the exception of psychotherapy and hypnosis, however, the focus in this chapter is on proven *self-care* approaches that you can begin using immediately to heal your mind along with your backache. They include *creating new beliefs and affirmations, establishing clear goals, guided imagery, visualization, breathwork, meditation, dreamwork, journaling,* and your approaches to both *work* and *play.* Each of these methods can help you become more aware of your habitual thoughts, attitudes, and emotions—both pleasurable and painful—in order to create a mindset conducive to experiencing optimal health and more effectively meeting your professional goals and personal desires, including freeing yourself from the restraints of disabling back pain.

THE MIND-BODY CONNECTION

Growing numbers of Western scientists and physicians now recognize that *body* and *mind* are not separate aspects of our being but interrelated expressions of the same experience. Their view is based on the findings of researchers working in the field of *psychoneuroimmunology* (PNI), also referred to as "neuroscience," which for the past three decades has shown us that our thoughts, emotions, and attitudes can directly influence immune and hormone function. In light of such research, scientists now commonly speak of the mind's ability to control the body. In large part, this perspective is due to the scientific discovery of "messenger" molecules known as "neuropeptides," chemicals that communicate our thoughts, emotions, attitudes, and beliefs to every cell in our body. In practical terms, this means that all of us are capable of both weakening and strengthening our immune system according to how we think and feel. Moreover, scientists have also proven that these messages can originate not only in the brain but also from every cell in our body. As a result of such studies, scientists now conclude that the immune system actually functions as a "circulating nervous system" that is actively and acutely attuned to our every thought and emotion.

Among the discoveries that have occurred in the field of PNI are the following:

- Feelings of loss and self-rejection can diminish immune function and contribute to a number of chronic disease conditions, including heart attack.
- Feelings of exhilaration and joy produce measurable levels of a neuropeptide identical to interleukin-2, a powerful anti-cancer drug that costs many thousands of dollars per injection.
- Feelings of peace and calm produce a chemical very similar to Valium, a popular tranquilizer.
- Depressive states negatively impact the immune system and increase the likelihood of illness.
- Chronic grief or a sense of loss can increase the likelihood of

cancer (and asthma, although this is my clinical observation and has not been scientifically documented).
- Anxiety and fear can trigger high blood pressure.
- Feelings of hostility, grief, depression, hopelessness, and isolation greatly increase the risk of heart attack.
- Repressed anger is a factor in causing many chronic ailments, including sinusitis, bronchitis, headaches, and candidiasis.
- Acknowledgment and expression of feelings strengthen immune responses.
- Anger decreases immunoglobulin A (a protective antibody) in saliva, while caring, compassion, humor, and laughter increase it.
- Chronic stress has a broad suppressive effect on immunity, including the depression of natural killer cells, which attack cancer cells.

As exciting as these discoveries are, the studies that had the greatest impact on me were performed on multiple-personality patients at the National Institutes of Health (NIH). Scientists found that in one personality, an individual could have the strongest possible skin reaction to an allergen or be severely nearsighted, but after shifting to another personality (an unconscious process in the *same* body) there was *no skin reaction* to the same allergen and perfectly normal *20/20 vision!* Science is just beginning to understand the depth and power of the connection between mind and body.

The implications of these discoveries are enormous and are producing a paradigmatic shift in physicians' approaches to treating chronic disease. They play an essential role in the Backache Survival Program: If emotions and attitudes can contribute to causing heart disease and cancer, it isn't too difficult to appreciate how they can also play a critical role in causing both acute and chronic low back pain. They are also tremendously empowering for anyone committed to holistic health.

Once you accept the fact that there is an ongoing, instant, and intimate communication occurring between your mind and your body via the mechanisms of neuropeptides, you can also see that the person best qualified to direct that communication in your own life is *you*. Learning how to do so effectively can enable you to become your own 24-hour-a-day healer by becoming more conscious of your thoughts and emotions and managing them better to improve all areas of your health. The first step in this process is acknowledging that you can no longer afford to continue feeding yourself the same limiting messages you most likely have been conditioned to accept since early childhood. Scientists now estimate that the average person has approximately 50,000 thoughts each day, yet 95 percent of them are the same as the ones he or she had the day before. Typically such thoughts are not only unconscious but often critical and limiting. For example, "I'm going to have to learn to live with this back pain [or any chronic condition] for the rest of my life." "I'll never get better." "I'll always be dependent on these drugs to relieve the pain." "I should've done _____ to prevent this situation." "I'll never be able to realize my greatest potential or fully enjoy my life as long as I'm stuck with this miserable _____." When you're hearing messages like these repeated many times during the course of a typical day, it's easy to understand why *fear, anger, hopelessness, sadness,* and *depression* may become the predominant feelings for people with a chronic condition like backache. You've just read that these painful emotions can be associated with weakening the immune system while also contributing to a myriad of physical problems. However, *by consciously taking control of your thoughts and recognizing how they govern your behavior, you can dramatically change your life and heal your dis-ease.* You will gain the freedom to think, feel, and believe as you choose, thereby flooding your body's cells with positive, life-affirming messages capable of contributing to your optimal health.

5. PLAY/PASSION/PURPOSE

The fifth item on my list of the *Essential 8 for Optimal Health* is a mental/emotional (and spiritual/social) health practice focused on living a life filled with passion. This requires a level of self-awareness that will allow you to better understand and appreciate yourself while recognizing:

- Your greatest talents and gifts
- What you most enjoy in life—what feels like play to you
- What would give your life greater meaning
- The purpose of your life—what you believe you came here to do

The next step on your path to optimal health is for you to begin creating a life that is more in accord with the responses to these self-posed questions. I've described this condition (holistic health) as the unlimited and unimpeded free flow of life force energy through your body, mind, and spirit. The remainder of this and the following chapter provide a variety of approaches to enhance this flow of life energy through your mind and spirit. They will provide you with valuable tools for gaining greater peace of mind, self-acceptance, and the self-esteem required to take the risks needed to proceed on your healing path, while enjoying more play and passion in your life. If you commit to diligently practicing one or more of these therapies, you will significantly reinforce and enhance the improvement you may have seen from the methods recommended in Chapter 4, and possibly cure yourself of backache.

BELIEFS, AFFIRMATIONS, GOALS, AND ATTITUDES

In his classic treatise *The Science of Mind,* noted spiritual teacher Ernest Holmes wrote, "Health and sickness are largely externalizations of our dominant mental and spiritual states. A normal healthy mind reflects itself in a healthy body, and conversely, an abnormal mental state expresses its corresponding condition in some physical condition." At the time Holmes wrote those words, in the mid-1920s, modern science was far behind him in understanding how *our thoughts directly influence our physical health.* But today a growing body of evidence not only verifies this fact but also indicates that our predominant, habitual beliefs determine the thoughts we primarily think. Socrates stated that the unexamined life was not worth living. Based on today's research in the field of behavioral medicine, we may paraphrase his statement to say, *"The unexamined belief is not worth believing in."* Yet most of us have never taken the time to actually examine the beliefs we hold. We therefore remain unaware of the extent to which they govern our behavior and how effectively they are currently serving us or affecting our state of well-being. Do most of your core beliefs, the majority of which you've held since childhood, reflect the truth of who you are today? If not, you can choose to replace them with those that do.

Beliefs

The importance of beliefs in the overall scheme of human functioning is confirmed by placebo studies. A "placebo" is a dummy medication or procedure that possesses no therapeutic properties and works only because of our belief in it. Detailed analysis of thirteen placebo studies from 1940 to 1979, including 1,200 patients, found an 82 percent improvement resulting from the use of medications or procedures that subsequently proved to be placebos.

Changing your beliefs is essential to your success with the Backache Survival Program. Most people suffering with chronic back pain have been told by their physicians: "You're probably going to have to learn to live with this problem"; "There's nothing more that can be done for you" (especially if you've already had surgery); or "There's no cure for your backache [or the majority of diseases]." These statements are, however, only beliefs. They are based on the limitations of modern medical science, a highly scientific and technologically advanced approach to the treatment of disease, and they are delivered to the patient by a highly educated individual in a society that defers to perceived expertise. These pronouncements, which are in some cases death sentences, are quickly accepted by most patients and become a part of their own belief system. The vast majority of people with terminal diseases who accept whatever their doctors tell them (these patients are called "compliant") die very close to their predicted life expectancy. By contrast, patients who challenge their physician's "death sentence" tend to survive much longer, and some of them go on to achieve full recoveries. In *Love, Medicine, and Miracles*, Bernie Siegel, M.D., vividly describes how the beliefs and attitudes of many of his cancer patients affected the outcome of their diseases.

Most of the beliefs held by Americans have been defined by the standards, or norms, of our parents and society, but how well does the norm fit for you today, as a unique adult? If all of us attempted to conform, the world would be a boring place, devoid of creativity and innovation. We certainly wouldn't be enjoying the ease of living that technology has provided us were it not for the adventurous few who deviated from the conventional belief system.

Unfortunately, in every culture there is great pressure to conform. It isn't easy, to say the least, to hold beliefs that run counter to prevalent attitudes. Family, friends, and society all tell us we have strayed, with phrases such as "You should . . . ," "You ought to . . . ," or—if your belief has caused them a lot of discomfort—"You're crazy!" Most of the time we respond to this pressure by giving up our unreasonable, or even outrageous, beliefs. Ultimately, almost all of us would prefer to be happy, accepted and loved by others, than fight for what we believe in or be proven right. Besides, we tell ourselves, "It wasn't that big a deal anyway."

Your belief system has a profound impact on your life: what your values and goals are; what you eat and think; how you dress and behave; what you do for a living; how you relate to others; who you choose to marry, befriend, or live with; how you spend your leisure time; and how you define health and quality of life. It also determines the nature of the silent messages you give yourself every day. All of us talk to ourselves, and this internal dialogue has a great deal to do with our state of mental health. These messages may be generally self-critical ("You stupid . . ." "Why did I say that?" "Why did I do that?" "How could I . . . ?" "I should've [could've] . . ."); limiting ("I'll never be able to . . ." "I can't trust anyone"); or accepting and supportive ("Good job!" "That's fine." "I did the best I could."). Almost all of my patients are very hard on themselves. They are self-critical and put themselves under a great deal of unnecessary pressure, while at the same time most are high achievers. As human beings we are imperfect; all of us make mistakes. The way we respond to these failings is what increases, or lessens, stress in our lives. Our pattern of response is one we probably have been repeating reflexively since childhood.

A very simple yet powerful exercise that can help you become more conscious of your thoughts, beliefs, and emotions is to devote 15 minutes to writing out all that you are thinking during that time. Do this when you are not likely to be disturbed—and don't edit anything out! After a few days of practicing this technique, many of your predominant beliefs will have been expressed on paper. Read them over. If they don't feel nurturing, build confidence and self-esteem, or regenerate and revitalize you, clearly they are not serving you and need to be either eliminated or changed. Pay particular attention to the *should*'s, *could*'s, and *never*'s. Before you discard what you write, examine your statements for possible clues to aspects of your life that may require more of your attention. For instance, if one of your statements reads, "I hate going to work," more than likely you may need to change your attitude about your job or leave it for one that is more fulfilling and better suited to your talents. (If the thought of leaving your job raises the thought, "How will I provide for myself and my family?" realize that this in itself can be a limiting thought. Numerous options will become available to you once you liberate yourself from your old assumptions and beliefs, whatever they may be.)

Affirmations

Once you have identified beliefs that are holding you back from your goals and desires or are negatively impacting your health, the next step is to begin to *reprogram* your mind with thoughts, ideas, and images more aligned with what you want. One of the most effective ways to do this is through the use of *affirmations,* or positive thoughts that you repeat to yourself, either verbally or in writing, in order to produce a specific outcome. Affirmations are positive statements repeated frequently, always in the present tense, containing only positive words, and serve as a response to an often-heard negative message or as an expression of a goal. For example, if some of the previous critical messages sound familiar to you, affirmations that would help counteract them are "I love and approve of myself"; "I am always doing the best I can"; "The world is safe and friendly." Even though they may run counter to your rational analytical mind, these positive thoughts create images that directly affect the unconscious, shaping patterns of thought to direct behavior and strongly impact outcomes. They act as powerful tools to unleash and stimulate the healing energy of love present in great abundance within each of us.

The purpose of affirmations is to replace habitual, limiting thought patterns and beliefs with more nurturing images of how you want your life to be. When affirmations are practiced regularly, they have the power to create optimal health by infusing the immune system with the life energy of *hope,* which triggers the activity of neuropeptides in the cells. Affirmations can be used to address virtually all aspects of your life, enhancing self-esteem, improving the quality of relationships, dealing with illness, and launching a more rewarding career.

Because of the simple nature of affirmations, the greatest challenge in using them is to suspend judgment long enough to allow them to produce the results you desire. When people begin repeating affirmations, they usually don't believe what they're saying (that's why they're saying them), although they would like to. Using affirmations is like reprogramming a computer. Your subconscious mind is the computer that has been receiving the same message for years—as the direct result of the thoughts and beliefs you have held for most, if not all, of your life. (They may have even been carried over from a past life, but that's a subject for another book.) It's not essential that you identify the origin of the beliefs that no longer serve you. What's important is that you commit to changing their input with new "software."

Most computers have a capacity for processing information far beyond the ability of the majority of computer operators to access it. Similarly, neuroscientists believe that the average person uses only 5 to 10 percent of his or her total brain capacity. As mentioned earlier, the average person has about fifty thousand thoughts every day, and it is estimated that 95 percent of them are the same ones he or she had the day before. Since your brain is hearing the same "program" repeated over and over again, it's no wonder you are able to realize only a small fraction of your (and your brain's) full potential. *Mental health will help to develop your creativity—you'll be re-creating yourself—while allowing you greater access to the parts of your brain that have been dormant.* It is in that re-creational process that you'll find an almost limitless supply of joy and passion. You'll also encounter a few strong doses of pain to help keep you on track.

The best time to say your affirmation is immediately following the negative message you repeatedly give yourself. When you're feeling the frustration of suffering with another episode of back pain and thinking to yourself, "This will never go away," you can follow that hopeless comment with the affirmation: "I am healing my back and getting stronger every day." Positive statements like this while you're in the midst of practicing stretching exercises, changing your diet and the way you breathe, taking the supplements, and following the rest of the Backache Survival Program not only will help you to feel a little better but also will increase your level of hope. And as your backaches diminish in frequency, duration, and/or intensity, you'll believe the affirmation more and more until it is actually true.

After you read "Emotional Causes of Backache" on page 205,

think about how the information regarding some of the more common emotional factors might relate to you. At the same time, you should also consider the content of your often-heard silent messages. If you find that one or more of these specific issues applies to you, then I would recommend creating affirmations to help lessen the harmful impact they might be having on your backache.

There are a variety of ways to use affirmations, although I've found from my personal experience and research on the subject that stating them verbally is most effective. Some people find that they get their best results by writing each affirmation ten to twenty times a day. Others prefer to say them out loud or to record them on to a cassette that they can then play back to themselves daily. One powerful technique suggested by Louise Hay, author of the best-selling *You Can Heal Your Life* (see page 206), is to stare into a mirror and make eye contact with your reflection while verbally repeating each affirmation. Hay notes that this experience tends to bring up feelings of discomfort at first and recommends that you continue the process until such feelings lessen or fade away altogether. You can experiment with these and other methods until you find the one that works best for you. Here are some other guidelines to ensure that you get the best results from your affirmation program:

(1) Always state your affirmation in the present tense and keep it positive. For example, if one of your goals is to be free of job-related stress, the affirmation *"I accomplish my daily responsibilities with ease and satisfaction"* will produce far more effective results than statements such as *"My job no longer makes me stressful."* The reason why affirmations work is because the unconscious accepts them as statements of fact and immediately begins to reorganize your life experience to match what you are telling it. So state *what you desire,* not what you wish to be free from, and write and say your affirmation in the present tense *as if your desire were already accomplished.*

(2) Keep your affirmations simple and short, no longer than two brief sentences.

(3) Say or write each affirmation at least ten to twenty times each day.

(4) Whenever you experience yourself thinking or hearing a habitual negative message, counteract it by focusing on your affirmation. Over time, you will find that your tendency to give yourself negative messages will diminish.

(5) Schedule a time each day to do your affirmations—and adhere to it. Doing something regularly at the same time each day adds to the momentum of what you are trying to achieve and eventually will become a positive, effortless habit.

(6) Repeat your affirmations in the first, second, and third person, using your name in each variation. Using affirmations in the first person addresses the mental conditioning you have given yourself, while affirmations in the second and third person helps to release the conditioning you may have been accepting from others. For example, if your name is Tom and one of your goals is to make more money, you might write: "I, Tom, am earning enough money to satisfy all my needs and desires." "You, Tom, are earning enough money to satisfy all your needs and desires." "He, Tom, is earning enough money to satisfy all his needs and desires." In each case, write out or repeat the affirmation ten times.

(7) Make a commitment to practice your affirmations for at least sixty days or until you begin experiencing the result you desire.

Goals

You can use affirmations to help change any belief that doesn't reflect the truth of who you are, to help you achieve any goal, and to create or re-create the life of your dreams. Most of my patients have come to me with one or more chronic physical and mental problem. Their objectives are clear: to stop living with chronic pain, to stop having sinus infections, to eliminate their dependence on antihistamines and inhalers for treating allergies or asthma, to have more energy, to suffer less anxiety, and so forth. After they have begun to see a definite improvement in their physical condition, which is usually after they have been working on the physical and environmental aspects of the specific holistic medical treatment program (Backache, Headache, Arthritis, Sinus, or Asthma Survival Program) for one to three months, I recommend that they create a "wish list" in the form of affirmations. The following is an extremely effective exercise for transforming your life and creating optimal mental health.

- *List your greatest talents and gifts.* You have several. These are things that are most special about you or that you do better than most other people. Ask yourself, "What do I most appreciate about myself?"
- *Next, list the things you most enjoy*—both activities and states of being—for example, "I really enjoy just being in the mountains or on a beach." There will be some overlap with your first list. Many of the activities you enjoy doing are the things you're best at.
- *Next, list the things that have the most meaning for you.* This is important, because if your goal doesn't meaningfully encompass more than one area of your life, or have benefit to others in some way, more than likely it is incomplete, and you will lack the passion necessary to commit to it. As you list the meaningful things in your life, you will more easily recognize the talents and activities you enjoy that are most worth your while.
- *Now make a wish list of all your goals or objectives in every realm of your life*—physical, environmental, mental, emotional, social, and spiritual. Physical and environmental goals can include recovering from illnesses or ailments, engaging in or mastering a particular physical activity (anything you've ever considered doing), or living or working in a certain place. Mental goals might address career plans, financial objectives, and any limiting beliefs that you'd like to change. Emotional goals have to do with feelings and self-esteem. Social goals are about your relationships with other people, while spiritual objectives have to do with your relationship with God or

Spirit. As you do this part of the exercise, ask yourself, "What does my ideal life look like?" "Where do I see myself three, five, or ten years from now?" "What is my purpose—what am I here to do?" Do *not* give yourself a time frame within which to attain any of these goals, and remember, it is *not* necessary to have a plan for getting there.

- *Next, reword all of your goals into affirmations.* For example, a goal might be "I'd like to be free of back pain." Some simple affirmations might be: *"My back is now completely healed"* or *"My backache is improving every day."* Then compile a list of about ten affirmations that address your most important goals and desires as well as the most limiting beliefs or critical messages that you'd like to change. As you'll read on the following pages, back pain is often triggered by a lack of support. Effective affirmations for backache might also include: *"I am loved and supported." "All of my needs are being met."*

- *Recite your entire list at least once a day, and whenever you hear a negative, limiting, or critical message, recite the one affirmation that corresponds to that message.* Or you can record them on to a cassette and listen to them in your own voice. Perhaps the most effective method for deriving benefit from affirmations is to *write, recite,* and *visualize* them (see "Guided Imagery and Visualization," page 210). Using this method, you would write down your affirmation while reciting it aloud, and then close your eyes and imagine what the affirmation looks and/or feels like, engaging as many of your senses as possible. If you can't picture it, it helps to *feel* your affirmations as you recite or write them, since this brings more energy to the experience. Make the process as vivid and real as possible.

I learned this technique from a patient, a man who owns an oil company and works part-time as a psychotherapist. He'd had a terrible case of chronic sinusitis for many years. In our second session, one month into the Sinus Survival Program, I presented this idea of changing some of his limiting, critical, or negative beliefs and clarifying his goals and objectives as a foundation for greater mental health. Shortly after this visit, he formulated a lengthy list of affirmations and goals. Once each day he recited every one of his new beliefs, then wrote them down on a sheet of paper, and after each one he closed his eyes and visualized what that desire or goal would look or feel like. When I next saw him, just over two months later, he told me that he had been repeating this procedure of reciting, writing, and visualizing for sixty consecutive days. He was thrilled to report to me that at least half of his affirmations and goals had already become realities, including healthy sinuses! He continues to practice this method (using new affirmations) along with the physical and environmental health recommendations that he had implemented at the outset of the program. It is now more than eight years since my third session with him. During that time he has had only two sinus infections, and his chronic sinusitis remains cured.

My patients' affirmation/goal lists provide a blueprint of our work together. The lists also become their personal vision and give direction to their own self-healing process. You must be able to clarify your desires to have any chance of obtaining them, and as you do this exercise, try to be as specific as possible. The next step is to believe, however minimally, that it is possible for you to meet these goals. The more you repeat the affirmations, the stronger your belief will become.

Attitudes

The third step in this formula for self-realization is *expectation*. (The first step is identifying what you want—*desire;* then, second, strengthening the *belief* that it's possible to realize that goal.) The stronger your belief and the more objectives you have already reached, the higher your level of expectation will be. After my chronic sinusitis was cured, I developed the belief that anything is possible, one that has helped me to realize other dreams. Whatever it is that you *desire,* as long as you *believe* it's possible, you can *expect* it to happen. It is not necessary to know how, or to have a definite plan. Just be patient and flexible and be willing to accept the path that presents itself and the result, even if the "package" in which your goal arrives is different from what you had envisioned. If your objectives are clear, your intuition will help you make the right decisions to get what you want. Remember that you can always choose what to believe. Rather than continuing with the attitude "I'll believe it when I see it," why not try "When I believe it, then I'll see it"? There's a good book on this subject by Paul Pearsall, Ph.D., entitled *Wishing Well.*

I've repeatedly seen this technique change lives in a variety of ways other than curing disease. My favorite example is a woman from Tennessee whom I was treating for chronic fatigue, allergies, and sinusitis. In the early years of my holistic practice, I worked with a number of patients long-distance over the phone, never actually meeting them in person. An RN in her fifties, she taught in a nursing school in a small town and had never married, although she wanted to. She had resisted putting marriage on her goal list because, as she explained to me, "I know all the eligible men in town and in my church, and there aren't any possible candidates." I convinced her to include it on her goal list, and her affirmation read simply: "I am happily married." Within a few months, she received a letter from a former professor of hers with whom she had a friendship years earlier. His wife had died the year before, and he wanted to visit his former student. Within months they were engaged, and a year after beginning her affirmation she was happily married. Her tears of joy over the phone and her gratitude left me in tears as well. We both felt as if we had experienced a miracle.

How you choose to see your backache or any other chronic condition can play a vital role in the way the disease affects you and whether or not it goes away. Some of the early reactions to a chronic or life-threatening disease are denial ("There must be some mistake"), anger and frustration ("Why me?" "What terrible luck"), self-pity ("I'll never be able to enjoy life again"), and resignation ("I'll just have to put up with it and continue to live this way for the rest of my life"). All of these are quite normal and understandable responses to something as devastating as an incurable condition. However, if you are interested in healing yourself, it is important to go beyond this point and look at your disease in a different light. According to Bernie Siegel, M.D., who contributed the following material to the book *Chop Wood, Carry Water,* you have several choices:

- *Accept your illness.* Being resigned to an illness can be destructive and can allow the illness to run your life, but accepting it allows energy to be freed for other things in your life.
- *See the illness as a source of growth.* If you begin to grow psychologically in response to the loss the illness has created in your life, then you don't need to have a physical illness anymore.
- *View your illness as a positive redirection in your life.* This means that you don't have to judge anything that happens to you. If you get fired from a job, for example, assume that you are being redirected toward something else you are supposed to be doing. Your entire life changes when you say that something is just a redirection. You are then at peace. Everything is O.K. and you can go on your way, knowing that the new direction is the one that is intrinsically right for you. After a while you begin to *feel* that this is true.
- *Death or recurrence of illness is no longer seen as synonymous with failure after the aforementioned steps are accomplished, but simply as further choices or steps.* If staying alive were your sole goal, you would have to be a failure, because you do have to die someday. However, when you begin to accept the inevitability of death and see that you have only a limited time, you begin to realize that you might as well enjoy the present to the best of your ability.
- *Learn self-love and peace of mind, and the body responds.* Your body gets "live" or "energy" messages when you say "I love myself." That's not the ego talking, it's self-esteem. It's as if someone else is loving you, saying that you are a worthwhile person, believing in you, and telling you that you are here to give something to the world. When you do that, your immune system says, "This person likes living; let's fight for his or her life."

- *Don't make physical change your sole goal.* Seek peace of mind, acceptance, and forgiveness. Learn to love. In the process, the disease won't be totally overlooked: It will be seen as one of the problems you are having, and perhaps one of your fears. If you learn about hope, love, acceptance, forgiveness, and peace of mind, the disease may go away in the process.
- *Achieve immortality through love.* The only way you can live forever is to love somebody. Then you can really leave a gift behind. When you live that way, as many people with physical illnesses do, it is even possible to decide when you die. You can say, "Thank you, I've used my body to its limit. I have loved as much as I possibly can, and I'm leaving at two o'clock today." And you go. Then maybe you have spent half an hour dying and the rest of your life living; but when these things are not done, you may spend a lot of your life dying, and only a little living.

I realize that you will not die from your backache, but each of these options for looking at physical illness can work for you as a form of preventive medicine. In my experience, incapacitating pain and imminent death have provided the greatest motivations for people to change, but why wait until you have reached that point of crisis?

EMOTIONAL CAUSES OF BACKACHE

Although nearly every case of backache can be traced to a physical factor (an injury or accident) that first triggered the pain, there is almost always a significant emotional cause(s) that had been present for some time prior to the onset of obvious pain. Many people suffering with backache are unaware of these painful emotions, while the majority who are, have made no connection between their painful feelings and aching backs. This aspect of the mind-body connection that focuses on the specific emotional issues contributing to chronic physical ailments is currently positioned on the leading edge of holistic medical research. It is an essential ingredient in our quest to address each of the causes of dis-ease and is a vital component of the Backache Survival Program. The more clearly each of these factors is identified, the more effectively each of us can assume greater responsibility for treating and healing ourselves, and our aching backs.

After thirty-five years of training and practicing medicine, I am convinced that emotional pain has more to do with the manifestation of physical pain than any other single cause. Ultimately, every painful feeling can be traced back to the perception of the loss of love, a thought that often originates from childhood trauma (physical and/or emotional). However, in my experience, the healing process seems to work best if you begin at a more superficial level and look at your current thoughts, beliefs, and emotions that may have contributed to your backache.

There are several pioneers in this field who have helped to expand my awareness of this exciting aspect of holistic medicine. Not surprisingly, each is a highly intuitive woman without an M.D. or D.O. after her name. Louise Hay, in her classic book, *You Can Heal Your Life,* states that the back "represents the support of life" and that the mental/emotional issues associated with low back pain are "fear of money; lack of financial support." The affirmation that she suggests for helping to heal the low back is, "I trust the process of life. All I need is always taken care of. I am safe." Carolyn Myss is a gifted medical intuitive who wrote *Anatomy of the Spirit.* Her work is largely based on the Ayurvedic chakra system. Each of the seven chakras (Sanskrit for "wheel") is a spinning energy center in the body, associated with specific organs or body parts along with different mental and emotional issues and colors. They also correlate to the location of the seven endocrine glands. Ayurveda, the traditional medicine of India for several thousand years, teaches that, if there is an obstruction or restriction in the flow of energy through a particular chakra, it can result in physical dysfunction of a body part corresponding to that chakra. The usual cause of this restricted flow of energy is an unexpressed painful emotion that is often present from early childhood. An episode of physical pain can be successfully (and often temporarily) treated with medication, but unless the underlying emotional cause is addressed there will usually be a recurrence of the pain.

Low back pain usually results from diminished energy in the root or first chakra and/or the sacral or second chakra. They often overlap. But generally very low back pain (including the tailbone) is associated primarily with the root chakra, while low back pain that's somewhat higher in the lumbar area is connected to the sacral chakra. The root chakra, located between the tailbone and the pubic bone, connects us to our bodies and the Earth and is a grounding energy whose color is red. It directs our most basic needs of survival, security, and safety. Other aspects of root chakra energy are the ability to provide for life's necessities, feeling at home, and social and familial law and order. It also has to do with our sense of belonging and tribal connections (to family, religious or support groups, community, and/or other men and women). In addition to backache, a weakness in this chakra can also be associated with increased fear and insecurity, depression, sciatica, varicose veins, rectal tumors, prostate cancer, or immune disorders.

The sacral or second chakra is located in the lower abdomen, approximately two to four finger-widths below the belly button. It is a center of creativity, emotions, and feminine energy and has an orange color. It is the center of the energy associated with relationship dynamics (usually female one-on-one relationships, such as female-male, female-female, mother-daughter), sexual and financial issues, victimization, and blame and guilt. In addition to low back pain and sciatica, the physical problems most often associated with this chakra are impotence and infertility, gynecologic and urinary problems, and constipation.

To apply the mind-body approach of the chakra system to treating your backache, you can try to identify which of these issues might apply to you. See if you can determine what you're holding on to so tightly that it has caused a contraction of your muscles to such a severe extent that you're in pain. One of my Healing Touch instructors, Janna Moll, also teaches Energetic Healing. She explains back pain in the following way:

What happens energetically is that congestion in the energy body [chakras] triggers a memory from the past. The back represents what is behind you, and often unseen. The body [muscles] tightens as a protection against identifying the real source of the pain. As the body tightens and "holds on," more congestion is formed. This becomes a cycle of pain creating more and more constriction. As the body pulls in energetically, pain intensifies. In order to stop this pain cycle the muscles must be convinced to "let go." For this reason pain medication and muscle relaxants will be a benefit only if used to break this cycle of constriction, and only work temporarily.

Most of the common drugs used for treating pain, however, will also further constrict the energy system, so it is recommended that Chinese herbs, homeopathics, teas, or other natural sources, such as hands-on healing or relaxation techniques, be substituted. Keep in mind it is the cycle of pain/constriction that needs to be addressed and not the pain itself. While addressing pain and muscle contractions, it is essential to look at the underlying issue causing the constriction of energy. In energetic terms, your back is your support system and holds your issues from the past, or what is behind you. As you begin to investigate the issues, your feelings, and your history of back pain (especially the first time you experienced it), you need to ask yourself, "How did I feel unsupported?" The introspective process may reveal to you that this is indeed an old pattern. This might become apparent either from similar situations that have occurred in your life or from your response to a current event. This congestion or constriction can have expression in one or more of the following aspects: mental, emotional, and/or spiritual.

When you deal with issues as they arise instead of pushing them back into the past (out of sight—out of mind) or dealing with them quickly and superficially, you actually strengthen the body's ability to remain balanced and clear. In doing so, you are preventing the need for the body to force your issues into the tissues (and cells). This eliminates the pain cycle and maintains a healthy and vibrant immune system.

In summary, if you're feeling stressed about basic safety and security issues, a sense of not belonging or not feeling grounded or connected to the Earth, your backache is probably associated with congestion in your root chakra. And if you're feeling significant guilt or blame, having difficulty expressing your creativity and emotions, having relationship problems with a woman, or having serious sexual or financial concerns, your back pain is most likely connected with your sacral chakra. I believe that by directly addressing and working on these emotional issues, clearing and balancing the energy system with the help of a Healing Touch or Energetic Healing practitioner, and following the recommendations in Chapter 4, most incidences of backache can be greatly diminished or eliminated.

PSYCHOTHERAPY

The field of psychotherapy, an outgrowth of the theories and discoveries of Sigmund Freud, continues to evolve more than a hundred years since its inception. In addition to the mental and emotional benefits commonly attributed to psychotherapy, a growing body of research has documented that physical benefits can also occur. For example, in a study conducted at the UCLA School of Medicine by the late Norman Cousins, a group of cancer patients receiving psychotherapy for 90 minutes a week showed dramatic improvement in their immune systems after only six weeks. During that same period the control group of other cancer patients who received no counseling showed no change in immune function whatsoever.

Psychotherapy, by its very nature, is not a self-care protocol but can be extremely valuable for individuals struggling with deep-rooted mental and emotional problems. The most popular forms of psychotherapy are *classical* or *Freudian psychoanalysis, Jungian psychoanalysis, family therapy, cognitive/behavioral therapy, brief/ solution-focused therapy,* and *humanistic/existential therapy.* Though they all share the same goal of helping patients achieve mental health, their approaches can vary widely.

If you feel that psychotherapy may help you, you will gain the most benefit by choosing the approach best suited to your specific needs and objectives. In addition, be aware that the work of psychotherapy is increasingly being conducted by nonpsychiatrists, including psychologists, social workers, and pastoral counselors. One of the reasons for this, perhaps, lies in the fact that many of today's patients seeing psychiatrists are given a psychiatric diagnosis (depressive, manic-depressive, obsessive-compulsive, etc.) and then treated with drugs, such as the antidepressant Prozac. This trend within psychiatry, a departure away from counseling and toward greater drug therapy, makes it a less desirable choice for someone interested in a holistic and self-care approach. While psychotherapeutic drugs can be effective at times, especially over the short term, each of the drugs commonly prescribed by psychiatrists has the potential to cause unpleasant side effects. Equally important, by focusing on treating psychological symptoms with drugs, many psychiatrists are depriving their patients of the opportunity to change their attitudes and behavior and to learn how to understand and grow from their emotional pain. Finally, whichever type of psychotherapist you choose, make sure that he or she is someone with whom you are comfortable. Psychotherapy can only be effective in a situation of trust, so you may wish to interview a number of therapists before making your choice.

Hypnosis is also a successful psychotherapeutic modality for treating backache.

GUIDED IMAGERY AND VISUALIZATION

Visualization is a skill that all of us have and one that we use every day. Most of the time, however, we do so unconsciously, such as when we daydream. The fifty thousand thoughts we have each and every day are often accompanied by inner pictures, or imagery, with corresponding emotions. Since the 1970s, researchers, physicians, and other health care professionals have been examining how to harness these mental images in order to use them consciously to create improved states of well-being. As a result of their efforts, thousands of individuals nationwide are learning how to use visualization and guided imagery to enhance their health. In many cases their outcomes have been astounding. Since 1971, radiation oncologist O. Carl Simonton, M.D., for instance, has been a pioneer in developing imagery as a self-care tool for cancer patients to use to bolster their response rate to traditional cancer treatments, with remarkable success. The first patient to whom he taught his techniques was a 61-year-old man who had been diagnosed with a "hopeless" case of throat cancer. In conjunction with his radiation treatments, the man spent 5 to 15 minutes three times a day imagining himself healthy. Within two months, he was completely cancer-free.

A similarly remarkable case is that of Garrett Porter, a patient of Patricia Norris, Ph.D., another leader in the field of guided imagery. Garrett was 9 years old and had been diagnosed with an inoperable brain tumor. Using biofeedback techniques in conjunction with imagery based on his favorite TV show, *Star Trek* (he pictured missiles striking and destroying his tumor), Garrett was able to completely reverse his condition within a year, with brain scans confirming his tumor's disappearance. He has subsequently written a book about his healing entitled *Why Me?*

Numerous studies also confirm the health benefits of imagery and visualization. For example, college volunteers who practiced imagery twice daily for six weeks experienced a marked increase in salivary immunoglobulin A, as compared to a control group who did not practice imagery. In another study, the well-known drop in helper T-immune cells in students facing the stress of final examinations was greatly reduced in a group utilizing relaxation and imagery each day for a month before exams. And patients scheduled for gall bladder surgery who listened to imagery tapes before and after their operations had less wound inflammation, lower cortisone levels, and less anxiety than did controls who were treated with comparable periods of quiet only.

Like most of the other therapies outlined in this chapter, one of the most exciting things about guided imagery and visualization is that both techniques are powerful self-healing tools that can be used to create positive change in almost any area of your life. In addition to its value in enhancing physical health, imagery can help you feel more peaceful and relaxed, assist you in further developing your creative talents, create more fulfillment in your relationships, improve your ability to achieve career goals, and dissolve negative habits or patterns. All that is necessary is a commitment to practice the techniques on a regular basis.

Guided imagery and visualization work to improve and maintain health because of their ability to directly affect our bodies at a cellular level, particularly with regard to neuropeptides. In addition, the use of imagery can often provide greater insight into causes and treatment for chronic conditions, guiding us toward the most personalized and effective solutions for our particular health problems. This occurs because our mental images are so deeply connected to our emotions, which, as I have previously discussed, are usually interconnected with the events in our lives. By using imagery, you can become better aware of what emotional issues may lie beneath the surface of your life and begin the process of healing them.

There are two types of guided imagery and visualization: *preselected,* or preconceived, images employed by you or your health care professional in order to address a specific problem and achieve a specific outcome, such as healing backache; and imagery that occurs *spontaneously* as you sit comfortably, eyes closed and breathing freely. Both forms have value, so try each of them and see which works best for you. What follows are two techniques you can use to make imagery a part of your Backache Survival Program. The first is a form of preselected guided imagery, while the latter is conducive for allowing spontaneous imagery to occur on its own.

The Remembrance Technique   This exercise can be adapted to improve issues or conditions in any area of your life. It's called the Remembrance Technique because in our core selves we are already whole, and, in many respects, healing is simply a remembrance of that state in order to reconnect with it. Begin this exercise by sitting comfortably in a chair or lying down in bed. Select a time and place when you will not be disturbed. Close your eyes and focus on your breathing. Take a few deep, unforced breaths to help you relax. With each inhalation, imagine that soothing, relaxing energy is flowing through all areas of your body. As you exhale, visualize the cares and concerns of the day gradually disappearing. Do this for 2 to 3 minutes, allowing your breath to carry you to a place of calm relaxation.

Now choose the issue you want to focus on for the rest of the exercise, and recall a time when the outcome you now desire was something you had already experienced. For example, if you have back pain, remember a time when you were in excellent health and never had the slightest worry (even in the deepest recesses of your mind) about the limitations imposed on your life by chronic and at times incapacitating back pain. Allow yourself to reexperience that time, using all of your senses to make what you are imagining as vivid as possible. Once you have reconnected to the experience, bring it into the present *as if it were actually happening now.* Stay with the experience for at least an additional 5 minutes, mentally affirming that you *are* experiencing the state you desire here in the present.

Another form of preselected imagery is to focus on an image of healthy, supple, relaxed muscles on either side of your spine in your low back, with the perfect level of tension to support your upright posture—neither too relaxed nor constricted; relaxed muscles lining the blood vessels, allowing for the optimum amount of oxygen and nutrients flowing through the bloodstream (these could be represented by a radiant white light) supplying all of the tissues in your low back. As you picture this, you are taking deep belly breaths and feeling all of your tight muscles relax. Prepare yourself in the same way I've described above—sitting, relaxed, and focused on breath. Even though this is a preselected image (like Garrett Porter's missiles striking his tumor), it can also be a dynamic process in which the image changes and evolves with each session of imagery. You might see a radiant white light filling every cell in the muscles, ligaments, bones, and nerves of your low back. Or, another time, you might picture a guardian angel or spirit guide gently and compassionately caressing your back. Allow your imagery to be creative without placing any restrictions upon it. There is no one correct image to use for healing backache. Whatever works for you and feels good is the "right" image.

Spontaneous Imagery In this exercise, instead of preselecting a specific outcome, you are going to allow your own unconscious to communicate with you through imagery about whatever situation in your life you choose to focus on. As in the preceding exercise, sit or lie down comfortably in a quiet place, close your eyes, and focus on your breath until you feel yourself settling into a deeper state of relaxation. Now focus on the physical problem you'd like to heal or the area in your life into which you desire to gain greater insight, allowing thoughts and images to freely and spontaneously emerge. Although you may have chosen your backache to focus on, you may be surprised by what you experience, but *don't judge it*. Trust that your unconscious knows what you most need to understand, and allow your imagery to lead you to that answer. Continue this exercise for 5 to 10 minutes, and when you complete it, write down what you experienced so that you can contemplate it for possible further insight.

As a variation on this exercise, you can first ask a question of yourself, such as "Why do I have back pain?" or "What do I have to learn from my backache?" and then see what image appears. From there, you may find yourself engaged in a dialogue between yourself and your unconscious that results in answers and solutions you did not know were possible.

When you first begin to practice mental imagery techniques, don't be discouraged if at first "nothing seems to be happening." As with any new skill, achieving results with imagery takes time. Remember that the language of your unconscious, like the symbolism of your dreams, is usually not literal or rational. It may take some time before you are able to grasp the messages of the images you perceive. Keeping a written log of your experience can make learning this new "language" easier.

BIOFEEDBACK AND RELAXATION

Learning and regularly practicing biofeedback or any of the relaxation approaches can result in a significant reduction in both severity and frequency of back pain. A biofeedback therapist acts as a coach to help you to master this potentially highly therapeutic technique.

The essence of *biofeedback* is to learn how to encounter stress without adverse physiologic effects, such as muscle tension, rapid heart rate and respiration, perspiration, or lowered body temperature. A typical course of biofeedback consists of eight to ten weekly 30- to 45-minute sessions. Learning to control body functions such as temperature occurs through *muscle relaxation,* which is achieved through progressive relaxation, visualization, and breathing techniques. Both techniques—biofeedback and progressive muscle relaxation—can be taught by a skilled practitioner and are not difficult to learn. However, the key to your success in preventing and treating your backache lies in the daily practice of these techniques. The practice sessions can be a few seconds or minutes long but have to be very frequent. A conscious effort is required in the first few weeks of training, but gradually these very brief relaxation techniques can become a subconscious habit. It can be quite helpful in relieving tension throughout the day, which in turn will reduce the frequency of backache.

OPTIMISM AND HUMOR

In the Bible it is written: "A cheerful heart is good medicine, but a downcast spirit dries up the bones" (Proverbs 17:22). Science is now beginning to verify this ancient truth, revealing that optimism and humor are integral factors in one's overall health, providing both physical and mental benefits. One of the most famous anecdotes illustrating this point concerns Norman Cousins, who, in his book *Anatomy of an Illness,* attributed his recovery from ankylosing spondylitis (a potentially crippling arthritic condition of the spine) to the many hours he spent watching Marx Brothers movies and reruns of *Candid Camera* while taking megadoses of vitamin C. The more he laughed, the more his pain diminished, until eventually his illness completely disappeared, never to return. Based on his experience with humor, Cousins went on to explore mind-body medicine at UCLA. Today a number of institutions such as the appropriately named Gesundheit Institute in Arlington, Virginia, founded and directed by Patch Adams, M.D., are studying the healing potential of humor.

Some of the most in-depth research in this area has been conducted by Robert Ornstein, Ph.D., and David Sobel, M.D., who presented their findings in their book *Healthy Pleasures.* They discovered that the people who are optimally healthy also tend to be optimistic and happy and possess the belief that things will work out no matter what their difficulties may be. Such people maintain a vital sense of humor about life and enjoy a good laugh, often at their own expense. According to Ornstein and Sobel, these people also expect good things from life, including being liked and respected by others, and experience pleasure in most of what they do. They are optimists, who usually look at stressful situations as temporary setbacks, specific to the immediate circumstance and due largely to external causes. Pessimists, when faced with life-challenging events, tend to think they will be permanent *("It's going to last forever")*, generalize the problem to their whole lives *("It's going to spoil everything")*, and blame themselves *("It's my fault")*. Recent research at the Mayo Clinic suggests that pessimism is a significant risk factor for early death. Over eight hundred patients were given a personality test that categorized them as optimistic, mixed, or pessimistic. After their health status was evaluated thirty years later, the pessimists had a significantly higher-than-expected death rate.

Optimistic people also tend to laugh a lot, something that most likely plays an important role in their health. Studies have shown that laughter can strengthen the immune system. One study, for instance, found that test subjects who watched videotapes of the comedian Richard Pryor produced increased levels of antibodies in their saliva. Furthermore, subjects in the study who said they frequently used humor to cope with life stress had consistently higher baseline levels of those antibodies that help to combat infections such as colds.

Hearty laughter is actually a form of gentle exercise, or "inner jogging." Describing the physiological effects of laughter, Ornstein and Sobel write:

> A robust laugh gives the muscles of your face, shoulders, diaphragm, and abdomen a good workout. With convulsive or side-splitting laughter, even your arm and leg muscles come into play. Your heart rate and blood pressure temporarily rise, breathing becomes faster and deeper, and oxygen surges through your bloodstream. A vigorous laugh can burn up as many calories per hour as brisk walking or cycling.
>
> The afterglow of a hearty laugh is positively relaxing. Blood pressure may temporarily fall, your muscles go limp, and you bask in a mild euphoria. Some researchers speculate that laughter triggers the release of endorphins, the brain's own opiates; this may account for the pain relief and euphoria that accompany laughter.

In short, laughter's benefits are many and profound. Unfortunately most of us don't laugh enough. One study found that young children laugh about 400 times a day, while the average adult laughs only 14 times. When the question posed to octogenarians is "If you had your life to live over again, what would you do differently?" the answer often is "I'd take life much less seriously." Comedian George Burns, who lived to be 100, wrote the book *Wisdom of the 90's* at age 95. He attributed his ability to laugh at himself as well as loving what he did for a living as the most important factors in his longevity.

Both optimism and a sense of humor are directly related to our beliefs. If you wish to become more optimistic and experience more humor and fun in your life, practice the exercises outlined in this chapter (especially affirmations and imagery). It may take time before you achieve the results you desire, but your commitment will prove well worth it and will impact your mood, mental health, and even survival. Nothing quite epitomizes the free flow of life force energy as does laughter, and all of us can stand to laugh much more than we do. Be advised, however: There is one side effect to this powerful form of self-healing—more pleasure.

EMOTIONAL HEALTH

The emotionally fit are able to identify their feelings and can express, fully experience, and accept them as well. I have heard contemporary American culture referred to as the "no-feeling" society. The feelings are certainly present, but, as a result of our lifestyle, we have constructed such formidable protective barriers around ourselves that to a great extent we have become unconscious of our feelings, especially the more uncomfortable ones.

There are many psychotherapists who believe that there are only two basic human emotions—love and fear. The so-called negative or painful emotions, such as anger, grief, anxiety, depression, envy, guilt, hatred, hostility, jealousy, loneliness, shame, and worry, are all expressions of fear. The feelings of acceptance, intimacy, joy, power, approval, and peacefulness are all aspects of love. The greater our degree of fear, the less capable we are of experiencing love.

With any chronic condition or illness, including backache, fear becomes the predominant emotion. When this occurs, your greatest liability is your *loss of love*—for yourself and those closest to you. It becomes a much greater challenge to nurture yourself and to feel fully alive when you're consumed with the anxiety and insecurity created by your ongoing physical discomfort and disability.

Some mental health professionals contend that there are four basic emotions: love or joy, sadness, anger, and fear. So at any given moment you're feeling either glad, sad, mad, or scared, or some combination of these. In our culture it is not socially acceptable to express most of the "negative" emotions, and men especially are not supposed to show signs of weakness or insecurity or to cry *("Big boys don't cry")*. The majority of us have learned to repress these feelings until we are unaware that we even have them. Society has helped us suppress our painful (negative) feelings by perpetuating the myth of an emotionally pain-free existence. The numerous ads in the media for analgesics to treat the pain of headaches and arthritis, and the common use of alcohol or drugs to dull the pain of an awkward social situation or personal crisis, give us the clear message that *not only is pain a bad thing, but life can be pain-free.*

If, however, we would spend less time avoiding emotional pain and instead focus our attention on it, accept it, and relax into it, the pain would diminish or even disappear. *If we continue to ignore and repress it, it often manifests itself as physical pain, illness, or disease.* Redford Williams, M.D., a researcher in behavioral medicine at the Duke University Medical Center, has gathered a wealth of data suggesting that chronic anger is so damaging to the body that it ranks with, or even exceeds, cigarette smoking, obesity, and a high-fat diet as a powerful risk factor for early death. Williams reported that people who scored high on a hostility scale as teenagers were much more likely than their more cheerful peers to have elevated cholesterol levels as adults, suggesting a link between unremitting anger and heart disease.

In another study, Dr. Mara Julius, an epidemiologist at the University of Michigan, analyzed the effects of chronic anger on women over a period of eighteen years. She found that women who had answered initial test questions with obvious signs of long-term, suppressed anger were three times more likely to have *died* during the study than those women who did not harbor such hostile feelings. Chronic sinusitis is usually associated with a tremendous amount of unexpressed anger, and I've also found it to be the primary trigger for most colds and sinus infections, as well as an important contributing factor to backache, headache, arthritis, and many other chronic conditions.

Clyde Reid is director of the Center for New Beginnings in Denver. In his insightful book *Celebrate the Temporary,* he says:

> Leaning into life's pain can also be a lifestyle, and is far more satisfying than the avoidance style. It requires small doses of plain courage to look pain in the eye, but it prepares you for more serious pain when it comes. In the meantime, all the energy expended to avoid pain is now available for the business of living.

I am not advocating that you seek out painful experiences, nor am I proposing that you endure prolonged or persistent pain. That is called suffering. Health and happiness do not have prerequisites that require you to suffer. Life is to be enjoyed, but the notion that it can be lived entirely without painful feelings is an unhealthy belief. Pain and joy are intertwined, and *the more you allow yourself to accept, embrace, and feel both pain and joy, the greater will be your sense of emotional health.*

Of the mental-emotional connection, Albert Ellis, a psychologist and the founder of the Institute for Rational-Emotive Therapy in New York City, has said that "virtually all 'emotionally disturbed' individuals actually think crookedly, magically, dogmatically, and unrealistically."

David D. Burns, M.D., a psychiatrist and author of *The Feeling Good Handbook,* writes:

> Certain kinds of negative thoughts make people unhappy. In fact, I believe that unhealthy, negative emotions—depression, anxiety, excessive anger, inappropriate guilt, etc.—are *always* caused by illogical, distorted thoughts, even if those thoughts may seem absolutely valid at the time. By learning to look at things more realistically, by getting rid of your distorted thinking patterns, you can break out of a bad mood, often in a short period of time, without having to rely on medication or prolonged psychotherapy.

Burns offers the following list of thought distortions:

- *All-or-nothing thinking.* You classify things into absolute, black-and-white categories.

- *Overgeneralization.* You view a single negative situation as a never-ending pattern of defeat.
- *Mental filtering.* You dwell on negatives and overlook positives.
- *Discounting the positive.* You insist that your accomplishments or positive qualities "don't count."
- *Magnification or minimization.* You either blow things out of proportion or shrink their importance inappropriately.
- *Making "should" statements.* You criticize yourself and others by using the terms *should, shouldn't, must, ought,* and *have to.*
- *Emotional reasoning.* You reason from how you feel. If you feel like an idiot, you assume you must be one. If you don't feel like doing something, you put it off.
- *Jumping to conclusions.* You "mind-read," assuming, without definite evidence of it, that people are reacting negatively to you. Or you "fortune-tell," arbitrarily predicting bad outcomes.
- *Labeling.* You identify with your shortcomings. Instead of saying, "I made a mistake," you tell yourself, "I'm such a jerk . . . a real loser."
- *Personalization and blame.* You blame yourself for something you weren't entirely responsible for, or you blame others and ignore the impact of your own attitudes or behavior.

As I've already said, negative thoughts and the feelings they engender contribute to physical illness. Insecurity, feelings of being unsupported or unsafe, a lack of belonging or a loss of connection to the Earth, as well as conflict in a relationship involving lost or withheld love and/or blame, guilt, sexual, and financial issues are experienced by most people with backache. These emotions are frequently associated with several of the thought distortions described above. These repeated thoughts will often trigger fear or anger that, if not safely expressed, can cause muscle tension and trigger back pain. Many of these same critical and limiting messages are also preventing you from achieving your goals and seeing your "wish list" become a reality. These theories of Drs. Ellis and Burns constitute the foundation of *cognitive psychotherapy*—the form of counseling I've found to be highly effective for many patients with backache.

One self-care approach you might try for gaining greater self-awareness is to attempt to identify the mental and emotional issues that may have contributed to your backache. Other than the concepts described on pages 207 to 209 related to the chakra system and energy healing, one method I've used with my patients for many years is to consider the possible benefits or secondary gain resulting from having this condition. They may not be readily apparent, but if you're open to this introspective exploration, you'll usually find some answers, however minimal, to the question, "What are the benefits of having this backache?" One possible result of having an incapacitating backache is that you get to rest and not do anything. Perhaps it is providing you a chance to slow down, to let go of control, to be cared for and feel supported, and to reflect on what's happening in your life and how you're feeling about it. Would you have been able to meet these personal needs if you were not disabled by the backache? Other possible gains may include "My wife (or husband) is more nurturing and pays more attention to me"; "I don't have to work or exercise"; "I'm no longer expected to perform (at work or sexually) at such a high level, and that has reduced a lot of pressure (stress)." Whether it's more attention, a need for nurturing or support, job dissatisfaction, healing a relationship, or some other unmet need, I believe there are almost always some secondary gains associated with every chronic condition. Since you did not respond preventively, in order to meet those unconscious needs, your body created an illness or an incapacitating pain.

If these not-so-subtle benefits can be understood and appreciated and you become more aware of what your needs and desires are, it will help considerably in identifying the emotional causes of your physical problem and allow you to work on resolving them. Once you have become aware of the issues, you can then begin expressing your emotions while addressing the unmet needs that your feelings have revealed. The process continues with acceptance: knowing that it's O.K. to feel whatever you're feeling. This healing process will not only lead you to emotional health but will also help you practice preventive medicine and take you a giant step closer to being free of your back-ache. Remember, a basic tenet of mind-body medicine is that *your core issues are held in your tissues.*

BREATHWORK AND MEDITATION

The benefits of learning to breathe properly and consciously (see "Breathing Exercises," pages 74–77) go far beyond the phys-ical. Proper breathing can also improve your mood, make you more mentally alert, and help you to become more aware of deeply held and often painful feelings. Most important, by work-ing with your breathing you can begin to heal the wounded, fearful, rejected, unnurtured, unloved, unacknowledged, discon-nected, and disowned parts of yourself and bring them into wholeness.

The primary reason that so many of us breathe unconsciously and inefficiently lies in the fact that our breathing process began traumatically at birth. We were forcibly expelled from the secu-rity of the womb and compelled to take our first breath on our own when we encountered the outside world. Often that first breath came as a harsh and unexpected shock, accompanied by pain and confusion. In order to suppress such pain, newborns typically follow their first inhalation by pausing and holding their breath for a moment as they struggle to make sense of their new environment. Today, a number of researchers in the field of mental health speculate that this first pause in our breath not only sets the stage for a lifetime of shallow, inefficient breathing but also conditions us to suppress our painful emotions instead of learning how to accept and relax into them. You can observe this pattern in yourself the next time you find yourself feeling shock, fear, pain, or worry. If you take a moment to observe yourself in the initial experience of such emotions, more than likely you will find that you are also holding your breath or breathing very shallowly, or perhaps even wheezing.

Breathwork, also known as "breath therapy," is a means of learning how to breathe consciously and fully in order to deal with emotional pain more effectively and healthfully. There are many approaches to breathwork, ranging from ancient breathing techniques found in the traditions of *yoga, tai chi,* and *qi gong* to modern-day methods such as *rebirthing* (also known as *conscious connected breathing*), developed by Leonard Orr, and *holotropic breathwork,* developed by Stanislav Grof. All of them have in common a focus on the breath and the ability to move energy through the body and connect you with suppressed emotions and limiting beliefs in order to heal them.

Most breathwork therapies use the technique pioneered by Leonard Orr. In connected breathing, each inhalation immediately follows the exhalation of the preceding breath without pause. (Typically we breathe unconsciously, pausing between inhalation and exhalation.) The pattern of respiration can vary according to technique. Sometimes it is rapid; sometimes it is deep, slow, and full. In addition, some approaches recommend breathing in and out through the mouth instead of the nose, and both abdominal and chest breathing can be used. In rebirthing, sometimes the therapy is performed in a tub or under water with the use of a snorkel, although this usually does not occur until the client has had a number of "dry" connected breathing sessions and has become comfortable with the movement of energy and the integration of emotions that commonly occur during the rebirthing process. Because of the emotional release that can result from breathwork, it is advisable to learn the techniques under the direction of a skilled breath therapist. Once you gain proficiency, however, you will have at your disposal a powerful self-healing technique that you can practice daily on your own.

Meditation also offers a multitude of emotional health benefits, as well as significant backache improvement. The regular practice of meditation is an effective self-care complement to all of the therapies recommended in Chapter 4. There are numerous meditation techniques, but all of them can be accurately described as conscious breathing methods. Meditation's many documented physiological benefits include improved relief from chronic pain and backache; increased immune function; reduced stress, including decreased levels of adrenaline, cortisone, and free radicals; increased oxygen intake; lowered blood pressure and heart rate; and a reduction of core body temperature, which has been linked to increased longevity. Among the psychological benefits of meditation are greater relaxation; improved focus on the present instead of regrets and worries about the past and future; enhanced creativity and cognitive functioning; heightened spiritual awareness (including insights leading to the healing of past emotional trauma); improved awareness and management of beliefs and emotions; and a greater compassion and recognition of oneself and others as parts of a greater whole.

The following is a simple meditation technique that utilizes breathing to promote mental calm. Select a quiet place and sit in a chair with your back straight and your feet on the floor. Close your eyes and begin abdominal or belly breathing, inhaling and exhaling through your nose at a rate of three to four full breaths (inhale and exhale) per minute. The object of this exercise is to stay focused on your breath, allowing whatever thoughts you have to come and go without being absorbed by them. Should you find your attention wandering, bring it back to your breath. You can also enhance the process by silently repeating a short affirmation or a positive word or phrase (called a "mantra"), such as *God, love,* or *peace,* or *I-am* or *as-is,* on both the inhale and the exhale. At first, try to do this exercise for 5 minutes once or twice a day, gradually working up to 20 minutes twice daily. Don't be discouraged if at first you find this exercise difficult to practice. For most Americans, sitting and breathing without thinking or external stimulation is not easy. With time and continued practice, especially in the morning and before you go to bed, you will begin to notice the benefits afforded by meditation. (For more on meditation, see Chapter 6.)

DEALING WITH ANGER

Unexpressed anger, or anger that is expressed inappropriately, is both harmful and extremely common in our society. Most of us were taught very early in life that anger was an unacceptable emotion. When it was expressed, it often elicited fear in us and was usually equated with bodily harm and loss of control ("He's really lost it"; "He's out of control"). This inability to safely express anger has been shown to produce many serious health consequences, from heart attacks to migraine headaches. I believe it is also a major contributor to backache. Today many psychotherapists are combining sound and body movement techniques to help their patients deal with their anger, finding that such approaches can be far more effective than simply talking about it. The following techniques can be safely employed by anyone to release the highly charged emotional energy of anger. They are most effective when employed regularly as preventive measures, instead of allowing anger to build up into a state of chronic, health-impacting tension, much less explosive rage.

Screaming   This is the most common anger-release technique due to the fact that all of us already know how to do it. In his novel *Tai-Pan,* author James Clavell wrote that the chieftains of ancient Scotland for centuries maintained the custom of "the screaming tree." From the time they entered adolescence, males of the clan were instructed to go into the forest and select a tree to which they could express their discontent. Then, whenever their troubles grew too great to otherwise deal with, they would go to the forest alone and scream with the tree as their witness until their emotions settled.

The value of screaming is no secret to young children, who commonly scream when they are greatly upset, only to exhibit a smiling face moments afterward. For adults, the biggest difficulty involved is finding a place to scream in privacy. Screaming when you are home alone, in the basement or closet, in the car with the windows up, or in a secluded spot outside are all possibilities. To get the most benefit, take a deep abdominal breath before you scream, and then direct the scream from your diaphragm or deep within your chest cavity, as this will protect your vocal cords. As you scream, slowly move your upper body from side to side or up and down. Usually, after two or three screams in succession, you will begin to feel much better.

The Angry Letter (Not Sent)   This technique is increasingly employed by therapists to help their clients release their anger. It involves writing a letter to the people with whom you are angry, listing all of the reasons why you are upset with them. As you write, allow yourself to express whatever comes to mind, no matter how harsh or offensive it may seem. Once the letter is written, read it over, and if anything else occurs to you that you wish to express, write that down too before signing it. Then either burn the letter or tear it up into small pieces.

Punching   Punching a bag, pillow, or sofa, or hitting them with a tennis racket or baseball bat, is another effective method of dissipating anger (although not advisable if you're in the midst of a severe backache). Remember to grunt or yell with each punch. A variation of this method is to take hold of a pillow and hit it against the floor, sofa, or wall. With either approach, it takes only a few moments before you will start to feel your anger transforming into satisfaction and even joy.

Simply venting anger, however, doesn't do the whole job. In fact, one study in April 1999 concluded that punching to release anger actually tends to increase and prolong feelings of hostility. Although this finding runs counter to my personal experience and that of many of my patients who have benefited from this practice, there are several additional steps that can be taken to release anger. You can start by recognizing that your anger may be the result of unreasonable or even irrational demands you've made on yourself or someone else and that by maintaining these demands you are hurting yourself with increased stress. It is therefore in your best interest to release the demands and let go of the anger.

Aerobic Exercise   This is another quick-fix method for dissipating anger, but only a low-impact form of exercise should be undertaken by people with backache (see page 153). If, however, you're especially enraged about a particular incident or situation, wait at least 20 minutes and take some deep breaths before beginning a strenuous workout. There can be a greater risk of heart attack associated with exercise *immediately* following emotional trauma.

Journaling This is also an effective means of releasing anger and is probably a bit safer than punching and/or exercise for people with backache. (This written technique and its benefits will be discussed in detail in the next section.)

Remember, anger in and of itself, is simply a natural emotion. It's only when it remains bottled up inside of us unexpressed that it becomes unhealthy. *Safely and appropriately expressing your anger in socially acceptable ways can dramatically improve the way you feel, both emotionally and physically.* If you are experiencing anger as a result of what someone else has said or done and the feeling persists as you've gotten "hooked in" and feel yourself (your body) holding on to it, then repeat to yourself, "This isn't about me." This practice creates some distance from what has occurred while preventing you from feeling responsibility or guilt for creating the situation. And in most of these instances the statement is true!

DREAMWORK AND JOURNALING

Dreams can play an important role in your healing journey. Serving as symbolic expressions of your inner emotional life, dreams often provide the clues you need to better understand your mental and emotional states as well as the guidance you may need to heal personal life situations. Sometimes dreams can also reveal how to heal physical disease conditions. This was illustrated in a dream of Alexander the Great, recounted in Pliny's *Natural History*. One of Alexander's friends, Ptolemaeus, was dying of a poisoned wound when Alexander dreamt of a dragon holding a plant in its mouth. The dragon said that the plant was the key to curing Ptolemaeus. Upon awakening, Alexander dispatched soldiers to the place he had seen in his dream. They returned with the plant, and, as the dream had predicted, Ptolemaeus, as well as many others of Alexander's troops suffering from similar wounds, was cured.

In American society, dreams are often overlooked or ignored, although researchers like Stephen LaBarge, Ph.D., have in recent decades done much to scientifically demonstrate their importance. The two biggest obstacles that prevent us from getting the most benefit from our dreams are that we either do not remember or quickly forget them, or we do not know how to interpret the symbolism and imagery that they contain. Dream recall, however, is a skill that anyone can develop with time and practice. One of the keys to dreamwork is to commit to focusing attention on your dreams. A deceptively simple way to do this is to tell yourself each night before you fall asleep that when you awaken you will remember what you dreamt during the night. At first you may not experience much success, but regular affirmation of this technique will instruct your unconscious to make your dreams recallable eventually.

As you start to remember your dreams, keep a pad and pencil or a tape recorder by your bed so that you can either write down or verbally record them immediately after you awaken. All of us dream an average of three to four times each night. With practice, many people who make the commitment to record and study their dreams are able to train themselves to spontaneously awaken after each dream cycle to record the gist of their dreams before settling back to sleep until after their next dream stage. Recording your dreams *immediately* after you awaken provides the best results, since dreams are quickly forgotten once you get out of bed and begin your day. Initially, you may only recall fragments of your dream experience. Don't be discouraged if this is the case. Over time, the regular recording of your dreams will begin to yield more details. In addition, after you have recorded your dreams for a few weeks or months, you will start to notice as you read over your dream diary how certain symbols and events tend to recur. Pay attention to such common themes: Usually they contain the most important messages that your dreams have for you.

Learning how to interpret the symbolism of your dreams

takes time and practice. Certain psychotherapists, especially those with a background in Jungian theory, are skilled in dream interpretation and can help you, and a number of books on the subject can also guide you. Bear in mind, however, that your dreams are highly personal, and although many dream symbols do seem to be common to what Jung called "the collective unconscious," there is no such thing as a standard for dream interpretation that will work for everyone. As the dreamer of your own life, you are ultimately the person best suited to appreciate your dreams and discern their deepest meanings. By taking the time to do so, you can improve your mental and emotional health immeasurably.

Journaling is another simple but very effective way to become more conscious of your mental and emotional life and to help you better express your feelings. For sufferers of backache, this is usually a safer method than punching or aerobic exercise for releasing anger. The practice of journaling entails keeping a written record of your thoughts, emotions, and any other daily experiences that you would like to understand better. Instead of recording your dreams, you will be keeping a journal of your waking activities. When journaling is done on a regular basis, it usually results in increased self-knowledge, often with insights that are both enlightening and enlivening. In a very real sense, journaling can help you become your own therapist and/or best friend: Instead of trying to express what you're feeling to someone else, through the process of journaling you tell it to yourself. The result is that your journal becomes your own emotional diary.

Many people who begin the practice of journaling are amazed to discover how the simple act of writing out one's daily experiences can lead to sudden and/or deeper insights into what they are feeling. Journaling can also help you become better aware of your beliefs, providing you with the opportunity to recognize and change those that may be limiting you. As you journal, you will also start to take more control over what you are thinking and feeling, becoming less reactive to your life experiences and more creative in your approaches to dealing with them. Journaling also makes communicating with yourself easier and allows greater clarity, since you are free from judgment or criticism from others. Your journal is for you alone and isn't meant to be shared. Nor do you have to worry about spelling or grammar.

A number of researchers, including James W. Pennebaker, Ph.D., author of the book *Opening Up,* have documented the benefits that journaling can provide by writing about upsetting or traumatic experiences. For people who have difficulty expressing their emotions, particularly those that are judged to be negative such as anger or fear, journaling can be especially valuable as a tool for self-healing. The results of a recent study measuring the effects of writing about stressful experiences on symptom reduction in patients with mild to moderate asthma and rheumatoid arthritis were published in the *Journal of the American Medical Association (JAMA)* in April 1999. The subjects in the study were asked to write about the most stressful event of their lives for 20 minutes for three consecutive days. They changed *nothing else* in their treatment regimen. Four months later, researchers found a marked improvement in lung function in the asthmatics and a significant reduction in the severity of disease in the arthritics. This landmark study is a clear demonstration of the therapeutic value of expressing emotions in treating a physical condition. Since most patients with backache don't have the opportunity to relate their feelings to their physicians, writing in a journal or writing unsent letters (see page 227) can be a highly effective self-care technique.

For best results, try to write in your journal around the same time each day. This will help make journaling a healthy habit. Just before you go to bed can be an ideal time for journaling. You can express the emotions that you've been containing all day and can provide resolution to the day's events prior to going to sleep.

Journaling and dreamwork will not only help you to heal mentally and emotionally (and physically) but also can open up new vistas of adventure that can last you a lifetime.

WORK AND PLAY

Do you enjoy your job? Does your work utilize your greatest talents? Is your job fulfilling and challenging? Sadly, for the majority of Americans, the answer to these questions is no. Recent studies reveal that an alarmingly high proportion of our society—nearly 70 percent of us—do not experience satisfaction from our jobs. Unfortunately, there is a significant price to be paid for not loving your work, both physiologically and psychologically. For example, in a study conducted by the Massachussetts Department of Health in the late 1980s, it was found that the two greatest risk factors for heart disease lie in one's self-happiness rating and the level of job satisfaction. Low scores in these two areas were shown to be better indicators of the likelihood for developing heart disease than high cholesterol, high blood pressure, obesity, and a sedentary lifestyle. No wonder, then, that in the United States more heart attacks occur on Monday morning around nine o'clock than any other time of the week.

Your job is a vital aspect of your mental health. If you find yourself working at a job that you do not enjoy, chances are that you continue to do so because of one or more of the following limiting beliefs: I don't have a choice; I need the money; I'll never be able to make enough money doing what I love; I have no idea what I'd enjoy doing or what my greatest talents are. By using the techniques outlined in this chapter, especially in the section "Beliefs, Affirmations, Goals, and Attitudes" (see page 192), you can begin to liberate yourself from these unhealthy beliefs. You'll discover that you are not bound to your job for life and that you do have the ability to find a more fulfilling job for which you are better suited. Each one of us is blessed with at least one God-given talent, and there is at least one activity that we enjoy doing that we do quite well. *That* is where you need to begin to investigate what your gifts are. Write down your talents as outlined in the goal-setting section on pages 199–201, followed by a list of activities you truly enjoy. Then brainstorm all the possible ways you can think of in which you can earn a living combining your talents with each of the activities you wrote down. List every idea that occurs to you, regardless of how ridiculous it may seem. As you continue to practice this exercise, you will have a much clearer idea of new job options. At the same time, acknowledge that you are seeking a greater level of fulfillment, are willing to change and take a risk, and are committed to begin the exploration that will lead you to work that you love doing. In the process, you may discover that your capabilities are limitless.

Even if you are fortunate to have a job you do enjoy, you may still be prey to another modern-day dis-ease, *workaholism*. According to the Economic Policy Institute in Washington, D.C., the majority of Americans are working longer and harder than they used to. Our yearly workload has increased by 158 hours, compared to that of twenty years ago, including longer commuting times and fewer paid holidays and vacation time. That's the equivalent of an extra month's work per year. The average workweek has risen to 46 hours, while Americans take less vacation time than any other industrialized nation. To counter this tendency, it is essential that you regularly engage in the counterbalance to work: *play.*

Many of us have unfortunately relegated play to childhood; yet play is a crucial aspect of mental health and is unrivaled as a means of expressing joy, passion, exhilaration, even ecstasy. The word "play" comes from the Middle Dutch *pleyen,* which means "to dance, leap for joy, and rejoice," all activities that suggest a vibrantly healthy mental state. "Play" has also been defined as any activity in which you lose track of time. Believing that play is not appropriate adult behavior is both limiting and unhealthy.

If your work involves your greatest talents and is something you truly enjoy doing, work and play for you can seem virtually indistinguishable. Even so, to optimize mental health, find at least one other activity to participate in, besides your work, that you can thoroughly enjoy. Such activities include sports, games, dance, and active creative pursuits such as playing a musical instrument, acting, singing, painting, crafts, or gardening. An activity in which you are of service to others is also a possibility.

Although many people derive great pleasure from playing cards or chess and other board games or from stamp or coin collecting, all of these are mental pursuits. To create a healthier balance, select activities that utilize your body, allow you to better express your feelings and creativity, and perhaps even bring you to a greater level of spiritual attunement. Ideally, the activity should be something so consuming and absorbing that it requires your total attention, providing a pleasurable escape from your normal tension, stress, and habitual thought patterns. Choose something that instinctively appeals to you and do it on a regular basis, for at least an hour three times a week. Be prepared to make mistakes and look silly. That's part of the risk, and the excitement, of doing something new. The more you commit to and practice whatever activity you choose, the better you'll become at it and the more you'll enjoy the benefits it provides.

We live in a society where work has become the greatest addiction, and the majority of us gauge our self-worth according to our achievements and net worth. For this reason alone, the importance of play cannot be overemphasized. All of us, for a short time at least, need to regularly let go of that responsible, mature, working-adult part of ourselves to reconnect with our woefully neglected playful "inner child."

SUMMARY

The biggest obstacles each of us must overcome in order to achieve optimal mental and emotional health are our largely unconscious denial and repression of emotional pain, and our limiting thoughts, beliefs, and attitudes, which, when combined, create our unhealthy behaviors. The tools in this chapter will enable you to heighten your awareness, allowing you to consciously transform your life in harmony with your greatest needs and desires. The more you practice the methods outlined here, the more profound the impact on your mental and emotional health, as well as your physical health and your backache. *You will become more conscious of your behavior and gain the freedom to choose how you wish to think, feel, and behave.* By letting go of your fear of experiencing life more fully, you can relax while embracing and accepting all of your thoughts, beliefs, and emotions. This will allow you the joy of realizing your life's goals and the exhilaration of the unimpeded free flow of life force energy. Remember, only through fully experiencing *both pain and joy* can you truly use your unique gifts and talents to thrive and fulfill your life purpose. And *if you can't feel it, you can't heal it.* This holds true for backaches, headaches, arthritis, sinusitis, heart problems, or any other chronic dis-ease. Your underlying emotional pain will be mirrored back to you with the ill health of your body and/or your mind. But so, too, will vitality and happiness reflect a condition of radiant health.

Chapter 6

HEALING YOUR SPIRIT

SPIRITUAL HEALTH

What profit does a man receive if he gains the whole world only to lose his soul?

MATTHEW 16:26

COMPONENTS OF SPIRITUAL HEALTH

Experience of unconditional love/absence of fear

- Soul awareness and a personal relationship with God or Spirit
- Trusting your intuition and a willingness to change
- Gratitude
- Creating a sacred space on a regular basis through prayer, meditation, walking in nature, observing a Sabbath day, or other rituals
- Sense of purpose
- Being present in every moment

The ultimate outcome of holistically healing ourselves is the recognition that we are truly spiritual beings, the heightened awareness of the transcendent power known as God or Spirit, and the joy that results from that enlightenment. By making the commitment to become spiritually healthy, we open ourselves to the underlying life force energy to which all religions refer and which is known in holistic medicine as *unconditional love.*

Learning to love yourself in body, mind, and spirit is also the simplest and most direct way to learn to love God. To heal yourself spiritually means developing a relationship with Spirit in your own life and attuning yourself to Its guidance in all aspects of your daily existence. By doing so, you will begin to experience a profound reduction in your feelings of fear and a greater capacity for loving yourself and others unconditionally. You will also become better able to identify your special talents and gifts and use them to fulfill your life's purpose *while fully experiencing the power of the present moment.*

In the deepest sense, all *dis-ease* can be seen as a disconnection between ourselves and Spirit, and a deprivation of love. From that perspective, spiritual health encompasses not only a conscious awareness of the Divine but also an intimate connection to ourselves and to our families, friends, and communities. Just as mental health encompasses emotional health, spiritual health embraces social health. You cannot have one without the other. This truth is illustrated in the lives of the world's great spiritual teachers, including Moses, Jesus, Mohammed, Krishna, and Buddha, all of whom remained closely connected to their communities throughout the course of their ministries. Despite the apparent differences in their instructions to us, at their core their messages are actually the same: *Place God first in all that you do, and love your neighbor as you love yourself.* As you reclaim your spiritual health, you fulfill their intention.

ACCESSING SPIRIT

Every advance in knowledge brings us face to face with the mystery of our own being. MAX PLANCK, FATHER OF QUANTUM PHYSICS

You may believe that you are incapable of experiencing Spirit in your life, but that is not the case. *Spirit is present in any moment when we feel profoundly alive.* During these special moments, our predominant emotions are exhilaration and joy. Not surprisingly, most people with backache or any other chronic ailment generally have a lack of joy in their lives. The late Jesuit priest and scientist Pierre Teilhard de Chardin described "joy" as "the most infallible sign of the presence of God." Usually these fleeting moments surprise us: Our perception of reality is suddenly free of our normal judgments and concerns. Time seems to slow as we lose ourselves in *pure awareness.* Examples of these moments include experiencing the birth of your child, special times spent with your beloved, being present at the death of someone you love, witnessing a sunset or sunrise, entering "the zone" while playing sports, and being in the presence of inspirational works of art. Such peak experiences can also occur unexpectedly and spontaneously during the course of your normal routine, sparked by something as innocuous as hearing your favorite song on the radio. For most of us, these moments may seem to be accidental occurrences.

The purpose of this chapter is to help make your encounters with Spirit a more frequent and conscious part of your life. As you learn to master the techniques that follow, recognize that Spirit operates in much the same fashion as subatomic particles: Both can be identified without being directly observed. Most often, and especially at the beginning of your spiritual journey, Spirit will be identified by the traces It leaves behind as It flows through you. With time and attention, each of us can deepen our perception of Spirit in our lives. Among the ways of doing so are *gratitude, prayer, meditation, intuition, working with spiritual counselors, spiritual practices,* and *reconnecting with nature and loved ones.*

ARE WE SPIRITUAL BEINGS?
THE NEAR-DEATH EXPERIENCE

Most of us spend our lives deluded by the belief that our traits, habits, and actions are the sum total of who we are. In actuality, these characteristic behaviors make up only our conscious personalities, or the sense of self that psychology refers to as "the ego." Our ego is the source of our thoughts, judgments, and comparisons, which usually are based on past experience or future concerns. Largely fear based, the ego diverts our attention from appreciating the reality that exists in the present moment. We live most of our waking hours in this ego state; yet, our true self, the soul (your individualized expression of Spirit), extends well beyond the limits of comprehension of the human intellect.

Letting go of the ego entails a surrender of mind and body that most of us equate with death. The thought of our death can be overpoweringly frightful. However, it is also one of the surest methods for reconnecting with our true spiritual natures. Every experience we have of transcendence and Spirit is also one in which we feel exhilarated and access a dimension of being beyond body and mind. If death is the freeing of our deeper self, or soul, from the physical plane, isn't it possible that it, too, can be an exhilarating experience? Certainly that is the report given by the vast majority of people who have had "near-death experiences." These episodes, also known as NDEs, involve people who were considered clinically dead in emergency or operating rooms, or at the scenes of accidents, and were subsequently resuscitated. In almost every case, these people report being totally aware of what was happening around them and could see their bodies as separate from themselves, while also experiencing profound feelings of peace and unconditional love. Most express a reluctance to leave the spiritual dimension to return to their bodies. They also later report much less fear of death and a greater appreciation of life.

The consistency of the reports of NDEs confirms the observation of many physicians and researchers who have scientifically studied the phenomenon of death and dying—that the soul remains intact beyond the death of the body. One of the leaders in this field is Elisabeth Kübler-Ross, M.D., who has pioneered this investigation for most of her professional career. After nearly thirty years of scientific research, she has concluded that "death does not exist . . . all that dies is a physical shell housing an immortal spirit." She also describes the time that we spend on earth as but a very brief part of our total existence and teaches that *to live well while we are here means to learn to love*—which is an active recognition, engagement, and appreciation of

Spirit in ourselves and others. In one of her studies of over two hundred people who had had a near-death experience, almost all reported that they went before God and were asked the question, "How have you expanded your ability to give and receive love while you were down there?"

Whether or not you choose to believe the data being gathered in the fields of thanatology (the study of death) and NDE, there is mounting evidence strongly suggesting the existence of Spirit beyond the realms of mind and body. Choosing to believe this theory can heighten your creativity, enhance your healing capacity, free you to realize your life's purpose, diminish the level of fear in your life, and release the self-imposed limitations of past traumas. By becoming more aware of your soul—that part of yourself that does not die—you will be better able to take risks and pursue the dreams of your life.

The terrorist attacks of September 11, 2001, to some extent provided our nation with a collective NDE. It could have been any one of us in the Twin Towers or on those planes. For me, as I expect for many of you, that day became the catalyst for a much more lucid vision of my purpose, my mission, what I came here to do during this very brief period of time that I'm alive. I realized more strongly than I ever have before that I'm here to teach a very simple truth: All that's needed to be happy, healthy, and to live our lives as a thrilling adventure, is to commit to mastering the art and practice of giving and receiving love. From my personal experience, I can unequivocally attest to the fact that it's a lot more fun than living in a survival mode. Each of us has a choice, and the option I'm offering in this and my other books is to learn to love your life and savor the joy of being alive, while choosing to see your pain—both physical, emotional, and spiritual—as an opportunity to fuel your journey as an evolving spiritual being.

I believe that we are 6 billion souls who have chosen to be here at this particular time in our planet's 4.5 billion-year history. For the past three thousand years we have been hearing essentially the same message from every great spiritual teacher—Moses, Jesus, Mohammed, Buddha, Martin Luther King, Jr., and countless others—love your neighbor as you love yourself; do unto others as you'd have them do unto you; we are all children of God, created in His/Her image; and the kingdom of God is within each one of us. How many times do we need to have this lesson repeated? As a species, we humans *(Homo sapiens)* sure are slow learners. After all, we've been failing the same exam for more than ten thousand years.

According to L. Robert Keck, Ph.D., M.Div, author of *Sacred Quest,* the collective Soul of humanity has entered a critical stage in our spiritual evolution. Keck has spent the bulk of his professional career working on and refining a method for researching the evolution of humanity's Soul, its content, and its periodic transformations. That method has become known as "deep value research." He believes that ten thousand years ago humanity's Soul went through its first major transformation. Apparently, it was time for us to grow up—out of our "childhood" epoch and into our "adolescent" epoch. The evolutionary purpose for this phase of our evolutionary journey appears to have been the development of our ego and mental capabilities.

Consequently, for ego differentiation, we separated and distinguished humanity from the rest of nature. That deep and organic reduction of the human/nature whole into separate and distinct pieces—humanity and nature—resulted in dividing our Soul along gender lines, sublimating the feminine and elevating the masculine. This Epoch II "adolescent" value system, therefore, became dominated by reductionism, patriarchy, hierarchy, a projection and externalization of power, and the need to exert control through rigid belief systems and the massive use of violence. And, as a consequence of that value system, our concept of the Divine/human relationship and our focus of worship switched to that of a transcendent, masculine, and heavenly God. This is the value system that has shaped and conditioned all of mainstream human cultures dominating the world today. The world we know has been the world of humanity's adolescent evolutionary epoch.

Today, however, humanity's Soul is being transformed—only the second such transformation in humanity's entire evolutionary history. Our fear-filled world of paradigm shifts is a world of chaos precisely because an old value system is dying, while an entirely new deep value system is being born. The emergent values that will reshape our very thinking, and certainly will cause major changes in every institution, are:

- A profound reconciliation with nature
- A rediscovery of the ubiquity of wholeness
- A maturation of our understanding of power
- The realization that Soul is in and of time

These values imply an evolutionary purpose of adult spiritual development—after epochs of a peaceful and nature-based childhood, and the ego and mental development of our adolescence. It appears that it is now, finally, time to get our act together in body, mind, and spirit. The very survival of our species is at stake.

Charles Darwin began the final sentence of his book, *The Origin of Species,* with these words: "There is a grandeur in this view of life . . ." Keck, however, suggests that,

> if there is a grandeur in considering the wonders of biological evolution, how much more grand it is to consider a picture big enough to encompass a holistic synthesis of physical, mental, and spiritual evolution. The territory of Soul is the grandest of the grand, for it is Soul that facilitates an oceanic view of life, a view of how all life is interconnected and interrelated. It is Soul that provides life's meaning and purpose. It is, indeed, Soul that gives us the very capacity to experience grandeur.

As we enter what Keck describes as Epoch III in our spiritual evolution, we need to prepare ourselves. Intensive training will be required in order to diminish the mounting fear and rise above the survival mode of existence in which an increasing number of sufferers of backache and other chronic conditions are living. The remainder of this chapter will provide you with many options to thrive and more fully experience the joy of simply being alive.

6. GRATITUDE/PRAYER/MEDITATION

I include *gratitude, prayer,* and *meditation* together as number 6 in my list of the "Essential 8 for Optimal Health," since they are so closely related. Most religious traditions prescribe specific prayers or grace before meals as a way of thanking God for our food and sustenance. As with other spiritual practices, there is something to be gained from these rituals or they wouldn't have survived for thousands of years. A sense of gratitude for all the other areas of our lives can elicit similar life-enhancing benefits.

GRATITUDE

Gratitude has been called the "Great Attitude." Although most of us tend to take our lives for granted, they are in fact a gift, and every day that we are alive, each of us receives many blessings. Even times of pain and fear, such as a particularly severe back-ache, can be seen as opportunities for growth for which we can be grateful. Acute low back pain can at times be so incapacitating that the sufferer feels as if he or she is dying or would like to die. Although this usually results in an increased level of general anxiety, it is possible for this individual to use these painful experiences to develop a far greater appreciation of life. By committing ourselves to becoming more aware of our blessings, we strengthen our connection with Spirit and are able to better recognize the wisdom and intelligence that underly all of creation.

Once we allow ourselves to appreciate the lessons presented during times of struggle or life crises, the brunt of the pain subsides and a state of inner peace follows. This is especially true of most chronic diseases, which can be seen as external reflections of inner (emotional and/or spiritual) pain. Typically, when people choose to focus consciously on the positives in their lives and express gratitude for them, additional positive things start to happen. For instance, while you're learning to live with your backache, suppose you spent time each day focusing on the blessings and the many pleasures your body has provided you in the past, along with the multitude of basic functions for which it still serves you well. These include the ability to enjoy breathing, eating, drinking, digesting, eliminating, exercising, and making love. Although you have a chronic physical problem, which at times is incapacitating, you've still retained the capacity to give and receive love, choose your beliefs and attitudes, as well as experience, express, and accept all of your feelings. In addition, this physical disability can serve as a powerful catalyst for your becoming better acquainted with your soul and Spirit. You may never have recognized the spiritual being that you truly are, or your purpose for being here, had you not been blessed with back pain. This may sound unreasonable or even irrational to you, but it was certainly helpful to me in curing my chronic sinusitis. For many years I suffered and felt as if I were cursed. I angrily asked of God, "Why me? What have I done to deserve this misery?" Yet now I can clearly see how this physical pain has so enriched my life. It's taught me how to give and receive love— to nurture my body, home and work environments, mind, emotional body, intimate relationships, and my soul. It's provided me with the training I might not have received otherwise, for the work I came here to do. Healing myself and teaching others to do the same for themselves has become my full-time job. I call it "training to thrive," and, at 56, I'm healthier and more fit physically, mentally, and spiritually than I've ever been. Who knows what my life would have been like had I not been blessed with sinusitis, or you with backache.

Gratitude can produce powerful feelings of joy and self-acceptance and is an attitude that anyone can choose to have, just as you can choose to see the glass half full or half empty. By focusing on what you do have, instead of what you lack, you feel a sense of abundance that makes your problems seem much less acute, and you are better able to let go of negative thoughts and attitudes. This usually isn't easy to do, especially if you are feeling a great deal of fear or anger. But if you make the effort to release these painful emotions and *choose the attitude of gratitude,* even for a moment, wonderful things can happen.

Like any habit, that of recognizing and acknowledging the

gifts in your life requires practice. One simple way to begin feeling grateful is the following visualization taught by Rabbi Mordecai Twerski, the spiritual leader of Denver's Hasidic community. As soon as you wake up each morning, before you get out of bed, close your eyes and picture a person, scene, or situation that makes you feel happy to be alive and for which you are still grateful. You never would have had that experience if you weren't alive, and by allowing yourself to reexperience it, you open yourself up to the awareness that something equally wonderful can happen today. Create the habit of practicing this visualization each morning upon awakening, and you will soon instill in yourself a new attitude of anticipation and appreciation for the day ahead.

Another way to cultivate feelings of gratitude is by making a *gratitude list*. This exercise is best performed before going to bed, as a way to detach yourself from any concerns or problems you may have, in order to appreciate the gifts and lessons that came your way during the day. Some people prefer to write out their list; others simply close their eyes and mentally review their day, making themselves aware of all the things that happened for which they feel grateful. Either way works well. Complete the exercise by praying silently, giving thanks for all that you experienced and learned that day.

By making gratitude a regular part of your daily experience, you set the stage for living more deeply connected to Spirit. In the process, your life will be transformed into an increasingly joyous adventure.

PRAYER

The most common form of spiritual exercise engaged in by most Americans is prayer. Nearly 90 percent of us pray, and 70 percent of us believe that prayer can lead to physical, emotional, and spiritual healing. Most people who pray have a greater sense of well-being than those who don't, and, when polled, the majority of people who pray say that through prayer they experience a sense of peace, receive answers to life issues, and have even felt divinely inspired or "led by God" to perform some specific action. Interestingly, people who experience a "sense of the Divine" during prayer also score the highest on ratings of general well-being and satisfaction with their lives.

In recent years, a great deal of scientific study has focused on the beneficial effects of prayer. Among the studies is one by the National Institute of Mental Health (NIMH) in 1994, which examined nearly three thousand North Carolinians and found that those who attended church weekly had 29 percent less risk of alcoholism than those who attended less frequently. In the same study, the risk of alcoholism decreased by 42 percent among those who prayed and read the Bible regularly. Another NIMH study conducted in the same year found that frequent churchgoers also had lower rates of depression and other mental problems.

A review of 212 medical studies examining the relationship between religious beliefs and health by Dale Matthews, M.D., associate professor of medicine at Georgetown University, found that 75 percent of the studies showed health benefits for those patients with "religious commitments." Among patients with hypertension, regular prayer reduced blood pressure in 50 percent of all cases.

Among the pioneers in the study of the physiological effects of prayer and meditation is Herbert Benson, M.D., a Harvard cardiologist. In 1968, Benson began studying people who regularly practiced transcendental meditation (TM). The subjects meditated by focusing on a mantra, such as *Om,* that had no apparent meaning to its user. Benson discovered that repetition of the mantra resulted in a lower metabolic rate, slower heart rate, lower blood pressure, and slower breathing. He dubbed this physiological effect the *relaxation response* (RR). Benson then turned his attention to Christians and Jews who prayed instead of meditating, instructing them to repeat religious phrases such as the first line of the Lord's Prayer, "Hail Mary, Full of Grace," "The Lord Is My Shepherd," or "Shalom." He found that all of the phrases produced the same relaxation response that was trig-

gered by meditation and that the degree of physiological benefit was determined by the degree of faith on the part of the person praying.

Since 1988, Benson and psychologist Jared Klass have been
conducting a series of programs at the Mind/Body Medical Institute at New England Deaconess Hospital, inviting priests,
rabbis, and ministers to investigate the spiritual and health implications of prayer. In their studies, Benson and Klass developed
a psychological scale for measuring spirituality. People who scored
high in spirituality—defined by Benson as a feeling that "there
is more than just you" and is not necessarily religious—also
scored higher in psychological health. They also:

- Were less likely to get sick and were better able to cope if
  they did
- Had fewer stress-related symptoms
- Gained the most from meditation training
- Showed the greatest rise on a life-purpose index
- Exhibited the sharpest drop in pain

To begin the practice of prayer, start with any prayer that you
are comfortable with or recall from your religious training as a
child. You can also use a favorite psalm or passage from the Bible
or a prayer book you find especially meaningful. In addition,
you can engage in personal prayer, talking to God as if you were
speaking to your best friend. State your need or concern and ask
for God's help. (It is more effective to pray for the peace that
would result from having what you desire than to pray for the
specific things themselves.)

In an experiment performed by the Spindrift organization in
Lansdale, Pennsylvania, the effectiveness of directed and nondirected prayer was tested. (Those practicing directed prayer have
a specific goal, image, or outcome in mind, while nondirected
prayer is an open-ended approach in which no specific outcome
is held in mind. The practitioner of nondirected prayer does not
attempt "to tell the universe what to do.") The results proved
conclusively that chances are much greater for attaining the de-

sired outcome when one prays for "what's best"—"Thy will be done." Whichever form of prayer you choose, try to establish a regular routine and repeat your prayer morning and night.

MEDITATION

In the West, meditation has primarily been studied for its mental, emotional, and physiological benefits, while in the East it has been used for thousands of years to still the mind in order to heighten awareness and contact soul and Spirit. During meditation, practitioners enter into a neutral emotional state, becoming a witness to their passing thoughts and feelings as they move into a state of heightened attention that can ultimately result in pure awareness.

As with prayer, there are many ways to meditate. Meditation can be performed while sitting or in a supine position, or while on the move—walking, jogging, and even during sports. What all forms of meditation have in common is a focusing on the breath and an emptying of the mind of thought. With regular practice, meditators typically report increased feelings of calm and peace, improved mental functioning and enhanced powers of concentration, and a deeper connection to Spirit, which is often perceived as a quiet, inner voice guiding them in their actions. Other reported benefits include increased equanimity toward, and detachment from, life events; increased energy and joy; feelings of bliss and ecstasy; and increased dream recall.

It is best to learn meditation under the guidance of a qualified instructor, but a variety of books and audiotapes are also available on the subject. The simplest method of meditation is to sit in a quiet place, resting comfortably in a chair, with your spine erect and your feet flat on the floor. Close your eyes and begin focusing on your breathing, keeping your awareness on each inhalation and exhalation. The practice is done using belly or abdominal breathing (see pages 74–77). To improve your concentration, you may wish to silently repeat the words "in" as you inhale and "out" as you exhale. Or you can repeat a word or mantra, such as *love, peace, God, Om,* or *Hu* (both latter terms are names for the Divine). Allow your thoughts to come and go without lingering on them, as if your awareness were a running stream and your thoughts were simply leaves floating by. At first you may feel deluged with thoughts. Each time you find yourself becoming distracted, simply bring your attention back to your breathing. Eventually you may notice longer periods of silence between each thought. It may take months to quiet your mind to this extent, but with consistent practice your meditation *will* become deeper and easier. Try to sit for at least 10 minutes once or twice a day, gradually working up to two 30-minute sessions per day. It's important to keep your practice regular and consistent, but don't force things. If you find yourself too distracted or pressed for time, end your session until next time instead of sitting restlessly.

Walking meditation is another form of meditation that in recent years has been popularized by the Buddhist monk Thich Nhat Hanh. This means of meditation is often suited for active people who find it difficult to sit still. The goal is to focus your attention in the present by focusing on each step you take, in tandem with your breathing. To enhance your experience, you can mentally repeat *With each step I take, I am fully present to my surroundings.* Over time, as you practice this form of meditation, don't be surprised if you find that it becomes more difficult to hurry. The more you focus on the present, the less consequence that time has as you discover how profound even a simple act such as walking can be.

INTUITION

As you progress on your healing journey, eventually you will find yourself being guided by your intuition, which is often experienced as an "inner nudge" or a "still, quiet voice" speaking from within. If you are not already aware of your intuitive messages, most likely it is because your intuition is having a tough time competing for your attention. Most of the inner messages you hear come from your ego and tend to be loud, self-centered, and fear-based. Intuitive messages, by contrast, come from the heart and are usually more subtle, compassionate, energizing, and enlivening.

In order to develop your sense of intuition, you will need to slow down, eliminate distractions, and do a lot less talking. The methods provided in this chapter can help you to do so. Slow, relaxing walks are another helpful way to make contact with this inner guidance. The next step is learning to recognize when your intuition is truly speaking to you and when it is not. Learning to discern the difference requires practice. One useful method for determining if the "voice" you hear is indeed your intuition is to notice how it feels. Often, intuitive messages occur accompanied by feelings of excitement or an unequivocal sense that acting upon them is "the right thing to do." People who haven't learned to trust their intuition often experience doubts or fears immediately following such feelings. "How can I be sure this is true?" "What if I'm wrong?" These and similar questions can quickly quash your inner guidance if you haven't learned to trust it.

To help you know if the messages you receive are in your best interest, experiment with the following exercise. Out loud, tell yourself something that you know to be true. As you do so, notice how you feel. Now state aloud something you know to be false. Again, notice how you feel. People practicing this exercise usually experience feelings of discomfort, confusion, even pain, in their bodies when they make the false statement, whereas they feel in alignment with the statement that is true. (Often the sensations occur in the area of the solar plexus, with false statements provoking queasy feelings or tension.)

Allowing yourself to be guided by your intuition is ultimately an act of faith. At first, learning to trust and act on the intuitive messages you receive will involve risk. The more trust you bring to your practice, however, the easier it will be to take action. Realize, too, that sometimes the results of following your intuition may be painful. Such times are not necessarily mistakes. They can be seen as lessons teaching you how to listen more effectively. Or they may be necessary to facilitate your growth and help you to better understand the higher purpose toward which Spirit is guiding you.

SPIRITUAL COUNSELORS

Due to the many uncertainties that can be part of the spiritual journey, you may consider working with a spiritual counselor, especially if you haven't been in the habit of listening to your intuition or need help in "tuning in" to Spirit. Just as you would visit a doctor to heal your physical body, or a psychotherapist to heal mental and emotional issues, spiritual counselors can help connect you to your spiritual core. The most common resources for spiritual counseling are priests, rabbis, ministers, and other clergy. Spiritual psychotherapists, medical intuitives, clairvoyants, spiritual healers or shamans, and medical astrologers can also be of great assistance. What these healers have in common is an ability to see beyond the boundaries of the five senses. Their services may include helping you to identify your life purpose, pointing out opportunities for your spiritual growth, or scanning your body's bioenergy field to diagnose the underlying cause of a particular health condition. Their primary value, however, lies in the assistance they can provide in helping you to appreciate the meaning and lessons of your daily life, especially those that are most painful.

Because of the lack of certification in these areas, you may need to rely on references from people you trust, experience some trial and error, and call upon your own intuition to find a spiritual counselor. Keep an open mind and see how you respond to the information provided. Some of these counselors are truly gifted and can provide you with information that can be a catalyst for transforming your life.

SPIRITUAL PRACTICES

Most of us have some sort of spiritual orientation, even if it is no more than what we received in childhood. Yet we often fail to realize how much some of these practices can contribute to our health. The ritual observance of *Sabbath,* for instance, can be an enormously healing experience, as it restores the sacred rhythm between work and rest. We're so busy *doing* in our society that we've forgotten how to just *be* and appreciate the delight of simply being alive. The Sabbath day is also a particularly good time to practice gratitude as you contemplate the blessings you share with those you love. Studies also reveal that those who regularly observe a weekly holy day tend to score higher in areas of optimism, stress management, and general well-being.

Fasting is another spiritual practice that is also healing. Not only can fasting have a cleansing effect upon the body, eliminating toxins while giving the organs of digestion and assimilation a rest, it can also elicit a heightened feeling of spirituality and result in the healing of old emotional wounds. In his book *Live Better Longer,* Joseph Dispenza, director of the Parcells Center in Santa Fe, New Mexico, points out that fasting can purge the emotional body of old, toxic feelings, facilitate the release of psychological patterns that no longer work for you, and "open your mind and heart to new emotional, psychological, and spiritual sustenance." (The Parcells Center is based on the work of Dr. Hazel Parcells, a scientist and naturopathic physician who, at age 41, cured herself of terminal tuberculosis using fasts and other natural methods. She then went on to live a life of vibrant, robust health until she died peacefully in her sleep at age 106.)

If you are new to fasting, try a 24-hour fast, selecting a day when work and other responsibilities are limited and you won't be too active. Plan for some quiet time alone, and, during the final two hours of the fast, drink six to eight glasses of water to help cleanse your body of toxins.

Gabriel Cousens, M.D., at his Tree of Life Rejuvenation Center in Patagonia, Arizona, has had great success in treating a variety of diseases, including arthritis, diabetes, asthma, and alcoholism, with fasting and meditation.

The following case history of a patient of my friend and colleague, Dr. Bob Anderson, clearly illustrates the healing potential of spiritual practices. Lois, a 64-year-old woman, underwent the surgical removal of a very large, aggressive ovarian cancer. The procedure left her with a colostomy, and part of the original tumor was not removable, leaving hundreds of small metastases throughout her abdominal cavity. On Dr. Anderson's insistence, Lois agreed to consult with an oncologist, only to promptly reject his recommendation of chemotherapy despite the fact that remnants of her tumor remained in her pelvis and abdomen. Convinced that her condition would be cured by her own body with God's help, Lois returned to Dr. Anderson to aid her in getting well. Although she undertook many initiatives, central to her program was her faith in the power of prayer and God. Each day she meditated for up to an hour and prayed numerous times.

Four months later, Lois was finally able to persuade her surgeon to remove the colostomy and thereby restore her internal bowel functioning. During the course of a long and tedious surgery, hundreds of small, metastasized tumors appeared as before. Seven of them were biopsied. Three days later, the pathology report showed that their cancerous characteristics were gone. Lois fully recovered and resumed an active life focused around the activities she enjoyed and her continued prayers to God. Two years later, an operation to repair an abdominal hernia revealed that her abdomen and pelvis were completely normal, without a trace of residual cancer. Although he has no way of proving it, Dr. Anderson remains convinced that Lois's daily prayers and meditations were somehow central to her recovery.

Finding Spirit in Nature

Nowhere is the creative power of Spirit more visible than in nature. It is here that we most directly experience life's four elemental forms of energy: earth, water, fire, and air. Earth is matter in its deepest form; water represents the receptive yielding principle; fire is the transformational energy that causes matter to change form; and air is the resultant blend of these other three elements into a subtler vibration of life force energy. In our bodies, earth is cellular matter, water is blood and circulation, fire is metabolism and energy production, and air is oxygen, the nutrient most essential to our sustenance. By regularly exposing yourself to nature's four elements—ideally, on a daily basis—you will expand your awareness of how each one is uniquely embodied within you and will more fully appreciate the healing power of nature. What follows are ways for you to do so.

Earth.   Spend as much time as possible outdoors in close contact with the earth. Walking is a wonderful way to do this, as are outdoor sports, bike rides in a park, and gardening. When you can, also visit the beach, woods, and mountains, and take time to notice the beauty surrounding you. The more time you spend immersed in nature, the more aware you will become of life's natural rhythms and the ways the earth retains and radiates energy.

As a society, we need to recognize that cities and other industrialized areas are in fact unnatural and can keep us from living a life of balance. Making the effort to spend time in nature can go a long way to restoring that balance while at the same time deepening your connection with Spirit.

Water.   One of the most visible forms of Spirit in nature is the flow of water as it follows the contours of the earth. Water is a receptive form of energy and is affected by the forces acting upon it. Rivers flow, for example, due to the gravitational pull caused by the gradient of the landscape. The action of water tumbling over rocks also releases a more subtle energy in the form of negative ions, which can contribute to feelings of well-being. Swimming in an ocean, lake, or river provides invaluable exposure to this special form of energy. Soaking in a mineral hot spring can also provide therapeutic benefits for a variety of ailments, especially backache, and can be one of life's great pleasures.

A healthy routine that anyone can adopt is bathing in warm water at least once a day. For added benefit, practice belly breathing while you enjoy a soak in the tub. This is a very effective way to connect with your body's bioenergy field and can help heal mental and emotional upsets. I strongly recommend soaking in hot water on a daily basis to all of my patients with backache.

Fire. Throughout the Bible and other sacred scriptures, the dominant symbols of the divine essence in human beings are fire and light, as in the tale of Moses speaking to God in the burning bush or the transfiguration of Jesus on the mountaintop before his closest apostles. Candlelight is also common as a tool for spiritual focus in most religions. Anyone who has experienced the pleasures of an open campfire can attest to the healing properties of fire. According to Leonard Orr, the founder of Rebirthing, spending time before an open fire, including a fireplace, cleanses the bioenergy field of negative energies and can be a powerful aid in curing physical disease. Orr recommends spending a few hours each day before fire for people who want to experience such benefits.

Fire is also an important component of the vision quests employed by Native Americans as a means of connecting to Spirit and discerning their life purpose. The ultimate source of fire energy is the sun, which provides healing and creative energy that directly or indirectly gives life to all living organisms. Regular exposure to sunlight has been linked to a variety of mental and emotional benefits, while depression, anxiety, and other mental dis-ease can occur when we are deprived of the sun's healing rays (for example, Seasonal Affective Disorder, or SAD). Time spent daily in the sun is a very healthy practice as long as appropriate precautions are taken, including sunscreen, hats, and long sleeves and pants when needed.

Air. Of the four elements, air is perhaps the closest expression of Spirit, so much so that the ancient Greeks equated Spirit *(pneuma)* with the wind. The most potent method of imbuing yourself with the life force energy of air is through meditation and other forms of conscious breathing.

A daily practice of exposing yourself to all four of these elements can significantly energize you, open you up to new levels of creativity and productivity, and make you more aware of Spirit's guidance and power flowing through you.

SOCIAL HEALTH

No man is an island.   JOHN DONNE

COMPONENTS OF SOCIAL HEALTH

Intimacy with a spouse or partner, relative, or close friend
- Effective communication
- Forgiveness
- Touch and/or physical intimacy on a daily basis
- Recreation
- Sense of belonging to a support group or community
- Selflessness and altruism

Our relationship with others is the crucible that most determines how spiritually healthy we are. *Optimal social health consists of a strong positive connection to others in community and family and intimacy with one or more people.* It is often much easier to feel our connection with Spirit during moments of solitude than it is to express that connection through our interactions with others. At the same time, our relationships offer us the greatest opportunities for spiritual growth and for experiencing unconditional love. *True spiritual health is a balance between the autonomy of the self and intimacy with others.*

The importance of social relationships, love, and intimacy with respect to health is documented in a growing number of studies demonstrating the benefits of the diversity and depth of connection to spouse, partner, family, and community. The lack of healthy social relationships is a common denominator among patients with heart disease, particularly when accompanied by feelings of hostility and a sense of isolation. Conversely, the longevity of terminal cancer patients with long-term survival rates has been attributed to a relatively high degree of social involvement. One of the most convincing studies highlighting the importance of community showed that Hispanics, despite poverty, lack of health insurance, and poor access to medical care, are surprisingly less likely than whites to die of major chronic diseases, including all forms of cancer, heart disease, and respiratory ailments. Further, with the exception of diabetes, liver disease, and homicide, their overall health outlook is significantly better than for whites. Some health experts, including former U.S. Surgeon General Antonia Coello Novello, the first Latina to serve in that post, postulate that the reason stems from Hispanic culture, which promotes strong family values and frowns on health risks such as drinking and smoking. Based on a growing number of relationship studies, researchers have concluded that *social isolation is statistically just as dangerous as smoking, high blood pressure, high cholesterol, obesity, or lack of exercise.*

The primary opportunities available to each of us for improving our social health include committed relationships and marriage, parenting, practicing forgiveness, friendships, selfless acts and altruism, and support groups.

7. INTIMACY AND CONNECTION–

Communication, Physical Intimacy/Touch, Recreation (CPR)

Committed Relationships and Marriage

Healthy committed relationships are probably the most effective and direct way to experience intimacy and unconditional love, in addition to promoting physical, emotional, and especially spiritual well-being. The model for all committed relationships is marriage, usually the most challenging as well as the most rewarding of all interpersonal relationships. It is potentially our most powerful spiritual practice. If humanity's fundamental moral principle is "Love thy neighbor as thyself," its practice begins not with the person living next door, but with the "neighbor" with whom we share our bed.

Regardless of who your partner may be or how long you have been involved with him or her, the key to all committed relationships is *intimacy*. Think of intimacy as *into-me-see*. As you develop the skills for seeing into—and learning to appreciate—yourself, you have the opportunity to also "see into" your partner and allow your partner to see into you. Once a commitment is made, the relationship becomes greater than the sum of its parts, allowing both partners to flourish and realize their full potential as human beings. The transformation that can occur in marriage and other committed relationships is primarily a result of letting go of judgment. As you do so, you will realize that, in giving more to the relationship, you are ultimately giving to yourself. Studies have shown that you may otherwise be contributing to making yourself and your partner sick. Marital conflict lowers immune function, especially in women, according to researchers at Ohio State University.

Hallmarks of a healthy committed relationship include *effective communication, physical intimacy* or *touch,* and *recreation.* My wife and I refer to them as "CPR for social health." Good communication encompasses the creation of a shared vision, attentive listening to each other, and the freedom to make requests so that both partners can better ensure that their needs are met. Regular intervals of fun and recreation together, along with daily doses of physical intimacy and touch, provide the glue for most thriving relationships. If you are interested in making a deeper commitment to your relationship, you might also consider working with a good marriage counselor or other relationship teacher.

Communicating

Shared Vision   A vision that you share with your partner is a way of defining your mutual goals and focusing your energy on their attainment. Lack of a vision can cause your relationship to lose direction or become stagnant. One simple but effective way to create a shared vision with your partner is to take time to individually list your relationship goals (keep them positive, short, descriptive, specific), prioritizing them in numerical order. Then begin combining lists, starting with the goals having the highest value and alternating between the two lists to form a composite vision that you and your partner are both comfortable with. The resulting "mutual relationship vision" can help keep you and your partner working together toward your common goals while reducing conflict and enhancing your relationship.

Attentive Listening   Most of us are poor listeners: We *hear* what is being said, but we don't always *listen* to it. This is because hearing can be unconscious, while listening requires conscious effort. Since communication is the foundation of any relationship and listening is a critical aspect of effective communication, it is important to get in the habit of consciously paying attention to what your partner tells you *without responding immediately.* The practice of listening can greatly enhance both intimacy and autonomy. This type of listening can be practiced as a "listening exercise." Schedule an uninterrupted 40-minute block of time in which you and your partner each speak for 20 minutes while the other person listens *without responding.* Talk only about yourself and how you're feeling, without blaming or talking about your relationship issues. There is no discussion following the exercise.

Attentive listening makes it possible for both partners to be able to talk freely and express thoughts and feelings without worrying about judgment or criticism. Focusing on what your partner is saying requires you to empty your mind of your own thoughts and concerns as you listen, thereby minimizing negative reactions. This exercise allows for a balance between intimacy and autonomy, a critical component of healthy relationships. Cultivating the habit of attentive listening will help you and your partner create a safe environment for expressing your feelings. This practice allows you to be more vulnerable and open with each other, which is extremely valuable for building trust, understanding, and deeper, even exhilarating, feelings of intimacy.

Requests By committing to another person, you enter into a relationship in which you have promised to give and receive love. But since each of us is different, what feels like love to one person may not even be noticed by another. Most of us attempt to love our partners in ways that feel like love to *us,* and are surprised when they do not react as we would. A good method for eliminating this problem is simply to tell each other what feels good to you and what you want.

It can be quite a revelation when someone you thought you knew well tells you what they really *need* from you. We often expect our partners to be able to read our minds, but we really can't know what the other wants unless we are told. Refrain from general statements such as "Love me" or "Be nice to me." Making specific requests like "I would like you to buy me flowers once a week" or "I would like you to cook dinner once a week" will significantly improve the likelihood that you will get what you need. When you do, be sure to thank your partner for complying with your request. This is extremely important, since your request is usually not an easy or natural thing for your partner to do. Otherwise, you probably wouldn't have had to ask for it in the first place.

Having Fun Together Life's daily pressures and responsibilities make it difficult to remember to have fun. For many couples, the glue that reinforces their relationship is the memory of the enjoyment they shared during their courtship and early years together. Setting aside time that you and your partner can spend in recreation together is an important way to *re-create* the joy and spontaneity that first brought you together. To rekindle some of that excitement and minimize the risk of boring routines, schedule fun activities together on a regular basis. Plan at least half a day each week to spend together away from home, taking turns each time to choose your activity. Getting out of the house, alone together, can help you focus attention on each other. Although this is more difficult to do if you have young children, it is still possible to plan an exciting evening at home after they go to bed. Choose something neither of you has tried before to add another dimension of adventure to your play, and, if you can manage it, plan several weekends per year out of town. This can be especially rewarding if a real vacation isn't feasible. Having fun regularly with the person you love is refreshing and invigorating and can help ensure that your relationship remains healthy and fulfilling.

Touch

Touch is not only one of our most effective healing modalities, it might well be the most powerful and direct means of conveying love. The lack of touch and physical affection is being recognized as a contributing factor in causing asthma, while massage has been shown to improve pulmonary function in children with asthma, as well as being effective in producing temporary relief of backache. According to Saul Schanberg, M.D., Ph.D., a professor of pharmacology and biological chemistry at Duke University, "Humans need to touch and be touched, just as we need food and water." His research and that of other experts were cited in *Hands-on Healing,* edited by John Feltman.

- In a study involving forty premature infants, half of them were gently stroked for three 10-minute periods a day for ten days; the other twenty were not. Although all were fed the same amount of calories, after ten days the touched babies gained an average of 47 percent more weight per day, were more active and alert, more responsive to social stimulation, and were able to leave the hospital an average of six days earlier than the untouched group.
- When a person's wrist is gently held by someone else, the heartbeat slows and blood pressure declines.
- Children and adolescents hospitalized for psychiatric problems show remarkable reductions in anxiety levels and positive changes in attitude when they receive a brief daily back rub.
- The arteries of rabbits fed a high-cholesterol diet and petted regularly had 60 percent less blockage than did the arteries of unpetted but similarly fed rabbits.

- Rats that were handled for 15 minutes a day during the first three weeks of their lives showed dramatically less cell deterioration and memory loss as they grew old, compared with nonhandled rats.
- In a study published in July 2000, Fijian women were found to have the lowest incidence of breast cancer compared to women from any other country in the world. This was attributed to the practice of breast massage which all Fijian girls are taught to perform on themselves as they reach child-bearing age.

Yet, in spite of the mounting evidence and healthy reasons to touch and be touched by other human beings (and, from the Fijian study, even by ourselves), Americans indulge very little in this simple pleasure. One study in the 1960s noted the number of touches exchanged by pairs of people sitting in coffee shops around the world. In San Juan, Puerto Rico, people touched 180 times an hour; in Paris, France, 110 times an hour; in Gainesville, Florida, 2 times an hour; and in London, England, the pairs never touched. The implications and possible causes of this phenomenon would entail a lengthy discussion, although I am sure the puritanical legacy of associating touch with sex has had a profound effect on American attitudes. William E. Whitehead, Ph.D., an associate professor of medical psychology at the Johns Hopkins University School of Medicine, believes that a significant part of the blame lies with the father of modern-day psychology, Sigmund Freud. According to Whitehead, "Freud encouraged austerity in dealing with children. And parents bought into that behavior." People who aren't cuddled a lot as kids, he adds, tend to develop into nontouching adults. The cycle then repeats itself, generation after generation.

As an osteopathic physician, I learned very early in my medical training about the therapeutic value of the "laying on of hands." Although almost all of our courses and textbooks were the same as those used to train allopathic medical doctors (M.D.s), we were also taught a holistic approach to health care that included osteopathic manipulative therapy. Soft-tissue stretching (somewhat similar to massage) and adjustments or corrections in the position of the spine and other body parts (similar to chiro-practic adjustments) are part of this therapy. It took me a while to realize that patients responded well to this treatment not only because of the prescribed techniques but also because of the healing potential of touch itself. It is now apparent that touch is helpful in treating backache (especially Healing Touch, massage therapy, and osteopathic and chiropractic manipulation) as well as most other chronic conditions.

There are a number of therapies in which touch is the pri-mary healing ingredient. They include acupressure, chiropractic, craniosacral therapy, Healing Touch, Hellerwork, various types of massage therapy, physical therapy, reflexology, Rolfing, Ther-apeutic Touch, and the Trager approach. Many of these were presented in Chapter 4 as being effective for treating back pain. If you are interested in experiencing a hands-on healing tech-nique, I suggest that you seek out the services of a practitioner of one of these therapies. And, if you're not so inclined, you can still enjoy the benefits of touch without visiting a professional practitioner. In a study demonstrating the benefits of massage on children with asthma, the parents performed the massage. I don't think most of us require a great deal of instruction on hugging or how to administer a loving touch. *Physical intimacy, including affection, strokes, and hugs, is a cornerstone of healthy relationships.*

Touching with love need not be sexual nor must it be given or received from another person to be beneficial. Animals are perfectly fine sources of tactile comfort, according to Alan M. Beck, Sc.D., the director of the Center for the Interaction of Animals and Society at the University of Pennsylvania. Numer-ous studies, he adds, "definitely show that petting an animal can lower one's blood pressure." Other doctors suggest that there are health benefits to be had even from cuddling inanimate objects—teddy bears, for instance. If you have neither a pet nor a favorite stuffed animal, my prescription for helping to main-tain your social health is to get several hugs daily!

There is no question that we have become too distant from one another. At a time when there are more of us than ever before (280 million), many holistic physicians and health care practitioners believe that *loneliness may be Americans' greatest health risk*. The recent trend toward more touching is our culture's attempt to restore a sense of wholeness and balance and to return to the norms and values of preindustrialized society. Most primitive cultures are very touch oriented. I have lived with one such native group in which touch is considered the traditional primary mode of healing. These people believe that their healers have a gift bestowed by God and that the healing energy that flows through the healer to the patient is God's love. Whatever its source, the healer's touch works quite well for a variety of ailments. By our standards these high-touch people might be considered primitive or underdeveloped, but they are clearly much healthier than most Americans in body, mind, and spirit.

Sex

Of all the major world religions, the Judeo-Christian tradition is the only one that does not commonly recognize the potential that sexual intercourse has as a pathway to Spirit. Other religions, including Hinduism, Buddhism, Islam, and Taoism, as well as the spiritual traditions of Africa and the Amerindians, freely acknowledge that sex, properly entered into, can be a powerful spiritual experience capable of transforming consciousness and enhancing physical and emotional health. In the West, perhaps the most well known of these teachings on sex is *tantra*. This is an ancient system of sexual and sensual techniques for consciously controlling the mind, increasing life force energy, and tapping into Spirit. Tantra's erotic practices include specific positions, breath, and visualization to heighten sexual energy and move it upward along the spine in order to create rapturous waves of blissful energy that can ultimately lead to enlightenment. Many mystic writings, such as the verse of the Sufi poet-saint Rumi, or the "Song of Solomon" in the Jewish/Christian tradition, also refer to the Divine using the language of sex and romantic love, often equating God with the Beloved while yearning to experience union with the Absolute.

To experience sex from this exalted perspective requires expanding your focus beyond physical gratification and genital orgasm into an experience of yourself and your spouse or lover as expressions of Spirit-in-the-flesh. Adopting this attitude leaves you extremely vulnerable and, simultaneously, in touch with your own divine power. Lovemaking in this state is free of the machinations of ego and proceeds slowly, gently, and consciously, ensuring that the needs of both partners are always met before moving on to the next cycle of pleasure and awareness. Couples who master this approach are able to remain in a state of heightened excitation for several hours, prolong and intensify orgasm, and experience total body orgasms. Among the experiences they report are a continuous flow of energy throughout their bodies, a joined climax of body and soul, and the sensation of being united with the cosmos and, afterward, being refreshed and revitalized. The primary goal of "spiritual sex" isn't prolonged orgasm, however, but an experience of being more deeply connected with the person you love and, through that connectedness, an awareness of your integral role within the whole of creation. Not everyone will feel the need to master, or even explore, a tantric approach to sex; yet all of us can benefit from more conscious lovemaking. Of all the spiritual practices, it is certainly the most pleasurable and potentially the most intimacy-enhancing. (To learn more about the tantric approach to sex, see *The Art of Sexual Ecstasy* by Margo Anand.)

Parenting

Parenting is easily one of life's most enriching experiences and, at the same time, one of the most challenging jobs. Through their children, parents have the opportunity to reconnect with play, to feel more in touch with their own "inner child," to experience selflessness, and to learn how to love unconditionally. Those of us who are parents are also provided with a wonderful forum for practicing forgiveness, trust, acceptance of ourselves and others, self-awareness, and, most of all, patience (as any parent of a teenager well knows). Perhaps the greatest human expression of love is that of parents for their children.

Unfortunately, in our society parenting isn't always consciously approached. If you are already a parent, however, it is not too late to meet your parental obligations more consciously than you may currently be doing. One useful guideline is to regularly ask yourself: *Will this [action, response, activity, demand] of mine help my child's self-esteem?* The same principle holds true in parenting as it does in marriage: *To love another is to help that person better love him- or herself.* This commitment will not only affect your child's happiness in the present but will significantly impact his or her future health. In the landmark Harvard Mastery of Stress study, college students rated their parents on their level of parental caring. Thirty-five years later, 87 percent of those who rated both parents low on parental love suffered from a chronic illness, whereas only 25 percent of those who rated both parents high in caring had a disease.

In the field of family therapy, the family is usually seen as a "system." This view holds that if a family member's behavior is harmful to himself or others, the problem and the solution lie not only within the individual but within the entire family system. This perspective encourages parents to examine their roles and the responsibility they share with their child for his or her problem. Often, a child's crisis serves as a mirror reflecting an imbalance in his or her individual system as well as in the family system as a whole. One of the significant advantages of family therapy is that change often occurs more rapidly than in individual psychotherapy. In much the same way that holistic medicine treats the entire person, not simply physical symptoms, the family-systems approach recognizes the need for family therapy when any family member is suffering—emotionally or physically. If this is a situation that applies to your family, family counseling is strongly recommended. The family-systems approach is practiced predominantly by social workers.

Good parenting requires both *time* and *consistency* in order to impart the values that you would like to instill in your children. Putting in time as a parent includes being with them on a regular basis and making an effort to get to know them better. What are their talents? What do they enjoy doing? What are they thinking about, and how do they feel? Learning the answers to such questions can pay big dividends for both you and your children. In fostering their growth as individuals, it is essential to give them greater power and responsibility by allowing them to make some of their own decisions. By permitting your children to participate to a greater extent in decision making, you will also instill confidence and trust, both in themselves and in you.

Other ways to spend time as a family are to worship together each week at church or synagogue and to designate a regularly scheduled time during the weekend for a fun activity. Take turns allowing each member to choose the activity for the day. It can be an effective confidence-builder. My adult daughters still talk about the family bike rides when, shortly after learning to ride two-wheelers, they would lead the four of us on a route of their choosing. The value of such play cannot be overemphasized. Having fun together as a family strengthens the bonds of love between each family member and defuses whatever stress or other problems may have built up during the week. Even if you cannot be with your children daily (due to being away on business or divorce, for instance), spending consistent time with them on a regular basis will help them experience the world and live their lives with the security, confidence, and caring that come from their knowing that you love them. Despite all of its inherent struggles and perils, parenting is first and foremost an incredible gift. Appreciating that gift by regularly interacting with your children is one of the most potent means that you will ever have for creating community and fostering both spiritual and social healing.

Friendship

A 1997 study from Carnegie Mellon University in Pittsburgh found that people with a greater diversity of relationships were less likely to get colds. Those with six or more social ties (family, friends, co-workers, neighbors, and so on) were four times *less* susceptible to colds than those with one to three types of relationships. Researchers found that it was not the number of people in the social network that was the important factor but the diversity. To varying degrees, most of these types of relationships can be called *friendships.*

As children and teenagers, most of us had a number of friends with whom we enjoyed sharing the day's adventures. Our friends helped us meet such challenges each new year as school, sports, puberty, dating, family problems, and the existential concerns through which all of us passed during our journey into adulthood. Between kindergarten and college, sustaining friendships was made easier by the fact that our friends provided us with a sense of belonging, a feeling of "being in this together," and offered us a forum in which to mutually discuss the problems and issues we faced at the time. Because of such friendships, many people regard the times they spent in high school and college as the happiest days of their lives. Once past college, as they entered the workforce, got married, and juggled the responsibilities of their careers and families, a large segment of our society has lost track of their friends from the past and have not replaced them with new friends.

While most adults enjoy the company of neighbors, co-workers, and other acquaintances, studies reveal that by the time we reach our thirties, those of us who still have a best friend in whom we can confide are exceptionally rare. This is particularly true of men who, because of this lack of a confidant, experience feelings of isolation and absence of support, no matter how fulfilled they may otherwise be in their personal lives and careers.

If you find yourself in need of a good friend, realize that it's never too late to rekindle old friendships or to make new ones. All that is required is a willingness to take risks and make the effort. Having a close friend you can talk to from your heart can provide many additional blessings in your life and deepen your connection with Spirit.

Support Groups

As a society we are plagued by social ills, most notably divorce rates that top 50 percent, a general sentiment of feeling overworked, dual-career marriages, increasing single-parent families, and a generation of children more adrift and alone than any that has preceded them. At the same time, a movement is afoot in America toward a greater sense of community in response to the silent epidemic of isolation and loneliness that affects so many of us. As a result, there has been a significant increase in support groups for those sharing common values, experiences, and goals. Support groups for couples, divorced people, single parents, men, women, people with an illness in common (especially cancer), and people recovering from alcohol and drug addiction—and other addictions—are gathering all over the country. Many of them are affiliated with a church or synagogue, with the added purpose of enhancing spiritual growth. They meet regularly—weekly, every other week, or every month—and the participants by and large report that they benefit from the social connection they find there. If you would like to participate in such a group, most likely you can find one in your local Yellow Pages, or you can contact organizations such as your local United Way, Catholic Charities, AA group, and the like. Many communities also have support groups devoted to specific diseases and can also be found on the Internet.

Recent scientific research also verifies that support groups can play an important role in helping people with chronic disease. David Spiegel, M.D., conducted a study at Stanford University School of Medicine on women with metastatic breast cancer. All of the women received chemotherapy or radiation therapy. One half of them were in a support group that met weekly for one year. These women lived twice as long as those who were not in a support group, and three were still alive ten years later.

Selfless Acts and Altruism

Remember a time when you stopped to spontaneously help someone, either a friend or a total stranger? Such selfless acts of giving go to the essence of Spirit, which is always with us, supporting our lives while asking for nothing in return. *Sharing* your time, help, and special gifts and talents with others in ways that benefit them provides you with an extremely effective means of engaging and expressing Spirit and enhancing social health. The opportunities for sharing are abundant and may include: donating clothes or money to worthy charities; volunteering time at a homeless shelter, soup kitchen, or after-school tutoring program; or simply setting aside personal tasks and concerns to address the needs of one's spouse or children. (There is a great deal of truth in the adage "Charity begins at home.") Another form of sharing that is regaining popularity is tithing. Dating back to biblical times, *tithing* is the practice of donating a certain percentage (usually 5 to 10 percent) of one's yearly income to charity. Interestingly, many people who adopt the practice of tithing also find that their incomes actually begin to increase, although that should not be your motivation for doing so. However you choose to perform selfless acts, remember that the truest form of giving is one that does not call attention to the giver. As Jesus instructed in the Gospel of Matthew, "When you give to the needy, do not announce it with trumpets." The purpose of sharing is *to share,* not to acquire praise or honors. Sharing selflessly will deepen your awareness of how abundantly Spirit is giving to you.

The late Hans Selye, a pioneer in modern stress research, thought that, by helping people, you earn their gratitude and affection and that the warmth that results protects against stress. Today, Selye's belief is borne out by mounting evidence that selfless acts not only feel good but also are healthy. Epidemiologist James House and his colleagues at the University of Michigan's Survey Research Center studied more than 2,700 men in Tecumseh, Michigan, for almost fourteen years to see how social relationships affected mortality rates. Those who did regular volunteer work had death rates two and one-half times lower than those who didn't. The highest form of selfishness is selflessness. When we freely choose to help others, we seem to get as much, or more, than what we give.

The closer our contact with those we help, the greater the benefits seem to be. Most of us need to feel that we matter to someone, a need that volunteer work can fulfill. There are a growing number of people requiring help in our society, including the homeless, the elderly, the hungry, runaways, orphans, and the illiterate, and there are many ways to help them. Choose to do so in the way that most compels you, but recognize that altruism works best when it comes from the heart and is not calculated as a means to receive something in return.

8. FORGIVENESS

To err is human; to forgive, divine.   ALEXANDER POPE

I have saved the most challenging but probably the most therapeutic of the "Essential 8 for Optimal Health" for last. The practice of forgiveness can generate profound health benefits. Intimate relationships and unconditional love cannot exist without forgiveness. How often do you blame yourself for your past actions and mistakes? How often do you blame others for your own problems, stress, or slights (both real and imagined) against you? Forgiveness cancels the demands that you or others *should* have done things differently. Hanging on to these demands changes nothing and keeps us under stress. Refusing to forgive yourself or others keeps you locked into limiting patterns from your past, unable to mobilize the creative power in your life here and now.

The next time you find yourself blaming others, physically point your index finger at them or their images and take a look at where the other three fingers of your hand are pointed. Right back at you! Forgiveness, therefore, begins with accepting responsibility for the role you play in shaping your life's experiences. Only after you begin to forgive yourself can you truly forgive others.

A key first step in your process of forgiveness is the recognition that you are always doing the best you can at any given moment, in accordance with your awareness at the time. This is true of everyone else as well. All of us make mistakes, and all of us ideally learn from them. You may even choose to believe that there are no mistakes, only lessons. In that moment, your action or behavior was based upon past experience, environment, and heredity. You can, however, consciously choose to be different in the future. To continue to blame yourself or someone else for something that occurred in the past is energy-depleting and keeps you from moving forward with your life.

Forgiving yourself may be your greatest challenge. No doubt there are a number of things in your past that you regret or for which you feel shame. (For me, parenting mistakes have been the most difficult to forgive.) But wouldn't it be healthier to look at what you can learn from your mistake or painful lesson so that it's not repeated; forgive yourself unconditionally for not knowing more or not performing well enough; and be grateful for this opportunity to learn to do better or change your behavior? A tennis player who misses a shot that he thinks he should have made will lose his confidence and ultimately his match if he doesn't quickly recognize what he did wrong, forgive himself, and move on to play the next point. Similarly, we lose the ability to focus and live up to our capabilities in the present if we do not forgive ourselves and let go of the past.

The more you are able to do this for yourself, the better you will be able to forgive others. *Remember, you are forgiving the actor, not the action.* You are not condoning cruelty, insensitivity, or incompetence; you are forgiving the offending person. By doing so, you are freeing yourself to move out of the past and into the healing present. Anger is the problem; forgiveness is the solution.

Bear in mind, however, that the people you decide to forgive may not choose to accept your forgiveness. Although their refusal to do so can be hurtful, their choice should be respected. What matters is that you are taking the step to heal the relationship. The act of forgiveness takes place within your own psyche, and the person you are forgiving may therefore be totally unaware of your action. Or you may be forgiving someone who is deceased. Be realistic and don't set your sights too high: Begin with someone who has been critical of you or guilty of another relatively minor offense. Forgiving others does not necessarily mean that your relationship with them will change, but forgiving them will enable you to feel a greater sense of wholeness. Your relationship with the people you forgive may remain the same on the surface, but it doesn't mean that healing hasn't taken place. You will know it when you feel it.

SUMMARY

Your spiritual well-being is ultimately the most important aspect of your ability to care for yourself. It is also the dimension of holistic medicine that is most often neglected in our society. Becoming spiritually healthy is a process of *diminishing fear and increasing love while developing an awareness of soul and Spirit and allowing It to guide you to a deeper connection to other human beings.* This infinite source of compassionate and forgiving transcendent power is the essence of all life on Earth and is the spark of life force energy within each of us. The most direct path to becoming spiritually healthy is learning to love yourself. As you do, you will appreciate the greater meaning and purpose of your life, experience gratitude for your many blessings, and become highly attuned to and trusting of your intuition. As you move beyond the confining restraints of your ego, you will become a more loving spouse or committed partner, parent, friend, and member of your community. In short, you will achieve the goal of holistic medicine: *to become whole,* and to experience a quality of life beyond anything you've probably ever imagined! Or at least beyond a score of 325 on the Wellness Self-Test.

REFERENCES

Acupuncture

Coan RM et al. The acupuncture treatment of low back pain: a randomized control study. *Am J Chin Med* 1980; 8(1–2): 181–85.

Ernst E, White AR. Acupuncture for low back pain. A meta-analysis of randomized controlled trials. *Arch Int Med* 1998; 158:2235–41.

Gunn CC et al. Dry needling of muscle motor points for chronic low back pain: a randomized clinical trial with long-term follow-up. *Spine* 1980; 5(3):279–91.

MacDonald A et al. Superficial acupuncture in the relief of chronic low back pain. *Ann R Coll Surg Engl* 1983; 65:44–46.

Van Tulder MW, Cherkin DC, et al. The effectiveness of acupuncture in the management of acute and chronic low back pain. A systematic review within the framework of the Cochrane collaboration back review group. *Spine* 1999; 24:1113–23.

Biofeedback

Schneider CJ. Cost-effectiveness of biofeedback and behavioral medicine treatments: a review of the literature. *Biofeedback Self Regul* 12(2):71–92.

Stuckey SJ et al. EMG biofeedback training, relaxation training, and placebo for the relief of chronic back pain. *Perceptual and Motor Skills* 1986; 63:1023–36.

Chiropractic

Cherkin DC et al. A comparison of physical therapy, chiropractic manipulation and provision of an educational booklet for the treatment of patients with low back pain. *N Engl J Med* 1998; 339(15):1021–29.

Coyer AB, Curwen IHM. Low back pain treated by manipulation: a controlled series. *Br Med J* 1955; 1:705–7.

Hadler NM et al. A benefit of spinal manipulation as adjunctive therapy for low back pain in a medical setting. *Spine* 1987; 12:703–6.

Meade TW et al. Low back pain of mechanical origin; randomised comparison of chiropractic and hospital outpatient treatment. *BMJ* 1990; 300(6737):1431–37.

Moore JS. *Chiropractic in America*. Baltimore, Md. Johns Hopkins University Press, 1993: 127–28.

Massage

Preyde M. Effectiveness of massage therapy for subacute low back pain: a randomized controlled trial. *CAMJ* 2000; 162: 1815–20.

Osteopathic Medicine

Andersson GBJ et al. A comparison of osteopathic spinal manipulation with standard care for patients with low back. *N Engl J Med* 1999; 341:1426–31.

Ernst E, Pittler MH. Experts' opinions on complementary/alternative therapies for low back pain. *J Manipulative Physiol Ther* 1999; 22(2):87–90.

Prolotherapy

Klein RG et al. A randomized double-blind trial of dextrose-glycerine-phenol injections for chronic low back pain. *J Spinal Disorders* Feb 1993; 6(1):23–33.

Ongley MJ et al. A new approach to the treatment of chronic low back pain. *Lancet* Jul 1987; 2(8851):143–46.

Yoga

Klein AC, Sobel D. *Backache Relief.* New American Library, 1985, New York.

Nespor K. Psychosomatics of back pain and the use of yoga. *Int J Psychosom* 1989; 36(1–4):72–78.

Telles S et al. Yoga for rehabilitation: an overview. *Indian J Med Sci* 1997; 51(4):123–27.

Miscellaneous

Cherkin DC, Eisenberg D, et al. Randomized trial comparing traditional Chinese medical, acupuncture, therapeutic massage, and self-care education for chronic low back pain. *Arch Int Med* 2001; 161:1081–88.

Jensen MC et al. Magnetic resonance imaging of the lumbar spine in people without back pain. *N Engl J Med* 1994; 331(2):69–73.

RESOURCE GUIDE

For more information about the Backache Survival Program or to make an appointment with Dr. Ivker, please call (303) 978-1474, or refer to the website: www.sinussurvival.com.

The following organizations offer additional information about various aspects of the Backache Survival Program and provide referrals to practitioners of the many therapies that contribute to this holistic approach for treating, preventing, and curing backache.

Acupuncture/Traditional Chinese Medicine

American Academy of Medical Acupuncture
4929 Wilshire Boulevard, Suite 428
Los Angeles, CA 90010
(323) 937–5514
Website: www.medicalacupuncture.org

Professional association of physician acupuncturists (M.D.s and D.O.s). Provides educational materials, postgraduate courses, and a nationwide membership directory.

American Association of Oriental Medicine
433 Front Street
Catasauqua, PA 18032
(888) 500-7999
Website: www.aaom.org

Professional association for non-M.D. acupuncturists. Offers publications and referral directory of members nationwide.

National Acupuncture Detoxification Association
P.O. Box 1927
Vancouver, WA 98668
(888) 765-NADA
Website: www.acudetox.com

Leading organization of its kind. Conducts research on and provides training in the use of acupuncture to treat addiction, including alcoholism.

National Commission for the Certification of Acupuncturists
P.O. Box 97075
Washington, DC 20090
(202) 232-1404

Provides information about acupuncture and offers a test used by various states to determine competency of acupuncture practitioners.

Qigong Institute/East-West Academy of Healing Arts
450 Sutter Street, Suite 916
San Francisco, CA 94108
(415) 788-2227

Provides education, training, and research about qigong in relation to health and healing.

Behavioral Medicine/Mind-Body Medicine

Association for Humanistic Psychology
45 Franklin Street, Suite 315
San Francisco, CA 94102
(415) 864-8850

Provides publications about humanistic psychology and a list of referrals.

Center for Mind-Body Medicine
5225 Connecticut Avenue NW, Suite 414
Washington, DC 20015
(202) 966-7338

An educational program for health and mental health professionals and laypeople interested in exploring their own capacities for self-knowledge and self-care. Provides educational and support groups for people with chronic illness, stress management groups, and training and programs in mind-body health care.

Mind/Body Medical Institute
New Deaconess Hospital
185 Pilgrim Road
Boston, MA 02215
(617) 632-9530

Provides research, training, and conferences related to behavioral medicine, stress reduction, yoga, and meditation.

National Institute for the Clinical Application
of Behavioral Medicine
P. O. Box 523
Mansfield Center, CT 06250
(860) 456-1153
Fax: (860) 423-4512

Provides conferences and information for practitioners.

Bodywork/Massage Therapies

American Massage Therapy Association
820 Davis Street, Suite 100
Evanston, IL 60201
(847) 864-0123
Website: www.amtamassage.org

Provides comprehensive information on most areas of bodywork and massage, including an extensive review of the latest scientific research. Also publishes Massage Therapy Journal, *available at most health food stores and many newsstands nationwide.*

Associated Bodywork and Massage Professionals
28677 Buffalo Park Road
Evergreen, CO 80439
(800) 458-2267
Website: www.abmp.com

Provides information and referrals.

Chiropractic

American Chiropractic Association
1701 Clarendon Boulevard
Arlington, VA 22209
(800) 986-4636
Website: www.acatoday.com

Professional association offering education and research into chiropractic. Also offers publications.

International Chiropractors Association
1110 North Glebe Road, Suite 1000
Arlington, VA 22201
(703) 528-5000
Website: www.chiropractic.org

Professional association offering education and research into chiropractic. Also offers publications.

Craniosacral Therapy

American CranioSacral Therapy Association
Upledger Institute
11211 Prosperity Farms Road
Palm Beach Gardens, FL 33410
(407) 622-4706
Website: www.upledger.com

Offers training, information, and referrals.

The Cranial Academy
8202 Clearvista Parkway, Suite 9-D
Indianapolis, IN 46256
(317) 594-0411
Website: www.cranialacademy.com

Provides information and a referral list of craniosacral therapists.

Diet and Nutrition

American College for Advancement in Medicine (ACAM)
23121 Verdugo Drive, Suite 204
Laguna Hills, CA 92653
(800) 532-3688

The ACAM provides information about the use of nutritional supplements and a referral directory of physicians worldwide who have been trained in nutritional medicine.

American College of Nutrition
722 Robert E. Lee Drive
Wilmington, NC 28480
(919) 452-1222

Information resource for nutrition research.

American Dietetic Association
216 West Jackson, Suite 800
Chicago, IL 60606
(312) 899-0040

Provides information and certification.

Center for Science in the Public Interest
1875 Connecticut Avenue NW, Suite 300
Washington, DC 20009
(202) 332-9110
Fax: (202) 265-4954

Provides a directory of organic mail-order suppliers, hormone-free beef suppliers, and general information on diet and nutrition.

Great Smokies Diagnostic Laboratory
63 Zillicoa Street
Asheville, NC 28801-1074
(800) 522-4762

Offers fully certified advanced assessments using over one hundred diagnostic tests of digestive, immune, endocrine, nutritional, and metabolic function—supported by a comprehensive network of educational and scientific resources.

International Association of Professional Natural Hygienists
Regency Health Resort and Spa
2000 South Ocean Drive
Hallandale, FL 33009
(305) 454-2220

Professional organization of physicians who specialize in therapeutic fasting.

Energy Medicine

International Society for the Study of Subtle Energies and Energy Medicine (ISSSEEM)
356 Goldco Circle
Golden, CO 80401
(303) 278-2228
Fax: (303) 279-3539

Research organization; provides education and information as well as publications.

Environmental Medicine

American Academy of Environmental Medicine
7701 E. Kellogg, Suite 625
Wichita, KS 67202
(316) 684-5500

Provides referral list of physicians practicing environmental medicine as well as a newsletter and other information.

Human Ecology Action League (HEAL)
P. O. Box 49126
Atlanta, GA 30359
(404) 248-1898

Provide referrals to support groups that assist people suffering from environmental illness.

Feldenkrais

Feldenkrais Guild of North America
3611 S.W. Hood Avenue, Suite 100
Portland, OR 97201
(800) 755-2118
Website: www.feldenkrais.com

Healing Touch

Healing Touch International
12477 W. Cedar Drive, Suite 202
Lakewood, CO 80228
(303) 989-7982
Website: www.healingtouch.net

Provides information and referrals.

Hellerwork

Hellerwork International
3435 M Street
Eureka, CA 95503
(800) 392-3900
Website: www.hellerwork.com

Herbal Medicine

American Botanical Council
P. O. Box 201660
Austin, TX 78720
(512) 331-8868

*A nonprofit research organization and education council that serves as
a clearing house of information for professionals and laypeople alike.*

Herb Research Foundation
1007 Pearl Street
Boulder, CO 80302
(303) 449-2265

*Provides research information and referrals to resources on botanical
medicine worldwide. Also publishes* HerbalGram.

Holistic Medicine

American Board of Holistic Medicine (ABHM)
1135 Makawao Avenue, #230
Makawao, HI 96978
(808) 281-5460
Website: www.amerboardholisticmed.org

The ABHM is the first organization to certify physicians in Holistic Medicine (December 2000 was the first certification examination) and to create the standard of care for holistic medical practice. Provides a referral list of board-certified holistic physicians (M.D.s and D.O.s).

American Holistic Medical Association (AHMA)
12101 Menaul Boulevard, NE, Suite C
Albuquerque, NM 87112
(505) 292-7788
Fax: (505) 293-7582
Website: www.holisticmedicine.org

The nation's oldest advocacy group (founded in 1978) devoted to promoting, teaching, and researching holistic medicine. Provides a list of referrals nationwide of holistic physicians (M.D.s and D.O.s) on its website.

Homeopathy

International Foundation for Homeopathy
2366 Eastlake Avenue East, Suite 301
Seattle, WA 98102
(206) 324-8230

Provides training in homeopathy and offers referrals.

National Center for Homeopathy
801 North Fairfax, Suite 306
Alexandria, VA 22314
(703) 548-7790

Offers training in homeopathy and provides referrals.

Medical Astrology

Jonathan Keyes
(503) 231-9146
Email: jonkeyes@qwest.net

Myotherapy

Bonnie Prudden Pain Erasure
P.O. Box 65240
Tucson, AZ 85719
(800) 221-4634
Website: www.bonnieprudden.com

Naturopathic Medicine

American Association of Naturopathic Physicians
2366 Eastlake Avenue East, Suite 322
Seattle, WA 98102
(206) 323-7610

Provides information, publications, and a referral directory of naturopathic physicians. Also in the forefront in licensing naturopaths throughout the United States.

The Institute for Naturopathic Medicine
66½ North State Street
Concord, NH 03301
(603) 255-8844

A nonprofit organization promoting research about naturopathy. Offers information to professional and laypeople, along with the general media.

Osteopathic Medicine

American Academy of Osteopathy
3500 DePauw Boulevard, Suite 1080
Indianapolis, IN 46268
(317) 879-1881
Website: www.academyofosteopathy.org

Affiliate organization representing D.O.s who provide osteopathic manipulative treatments and/or cranial osteopathy as part of their practice.

Reflexology

International Institute of Reflexology
5650 First Avenue North
P. O. Box 12462
St. Petersburg, FL 33733
(727) 343-4811
Website: www.reflexology-usa.net

Provides information, training, and referrals.

Reiki

International Center for Reiki Training
29209 Northwestern Highway, Suite 592
Southfield, MI 48034
(800) 332-8112
Website: www.reiki.org

Provides information and referrals.

Rolfing

International Rolf Institute
205 Canyon Road
Boulder, CO 80306
(303) 449-5903
Website: www.rolf.org

Provides information, training and referral directory.

Therapeutic Touch

Nurse Healers Professional Associates, Inc.
1211 Locust Street
Philadelphia, PA 19107
(215) 545-8079

Provides information on training, conferences, and referrals of Therapeutic Touch practitioners. Also publishes a newsletter.

Trager

The Trager Institute
3800 Park East Drive, Suite 100, Room 1
Beachwood, OH 44122
(216) 896-9383
Website: www.trager.com

PRODUCT INDEX

All of the following are available through Sinus Survival Services at 1-888-434-0033.

Products to Assist in Implementing the Backache Survival Program

Glucosamine Intensive CarePlus—glucosamine sulfate and chondroitin sulfate

Collagen Support—collagen

Super Potency Essential Fatty Acids—omega-3 oils, EPA, and DHA

Calcium Supreme—high-quality calcium (microcrystalline hydroxyapatite) containing glucosamine

Herbal Joint Relief—boswella, curcumin, and ginger

Herbal Muscle Relief—magnesium, calcium, valerian, and passionflower

Other Sinus Survival Products

Sinus Survival Masquelier's OPC Grape Seed

Sinus Survival Eucalyptus Spray

Professional Health Products Mycological Immune Stimulator

Sinus Survival Nasal Spray

Product Index

Kaz TheraStream Personal Steam Inhaler
SinuCleanse Irrigation System
SinuCleanse Saline Refills
Grossan Nasal Irrigator
Hydro-Pulse® Nasal Irrigator
Sinus Survival Air Vitalizer Ionizer
Bionaire ULPA Filter Air Cleaners
Bionaire ULPA Filter Replacements
Bionaire Warm-Mist Humidifiers
DuPont Vacuum Bags
DuPont Wizard Dust Cloths

BIBLIOGRAPHY

Anand, Margo. *The Art of Sexual Ecstasy.* Tarcher, 1989.

Anderson, Robert. *Clinician's Guide to Holistic Medicine.* McGraw-Hill, 2001.

————. *The Scientific Basis for Holistic Medicine.* American Health Press, 2001.

Borysenko, Joan. *Minding the Body, Mending the Mind.* Bantam Books, 1987.

Brownstein, Art. *Healing Back Pain Naturally.* Harbor Press, 1999.

Golan, Ralph. *Optimal Wellness.* Ballantine, 1995.

Goleman, Dan; Griffin, Joel. *Mind Body Medicine.* Consumer Reports Books, 1993.

Grimes, Carl. *Starting Points for a Healthy Habitat.* GMC Media, 1999.

Hale, Teresa. *Breathing Free.* Three Rivers Press, 1999.

Hay, Louise. *You Can Heal Your Life.* Hay House, 1984.

Hendrix, Harville. *Getting the Love You Want: A Guide for Couples.* Harper & Row, 1988.

Ivker, Robert. *Sinus Survival: The Holistic Medical Treatment for Sinusitis, Allergies, & Colds,* 4th ed. Tarcher/Putnam, 2000.

Ivker, Robert; Nelson, Todd. *Arthritis Survival: The Holistic Medical Treatment for Osteoarthritis.* Tarcher/Putnam, 2001.

————. *Asthma Survival: The Holistic Medical Treatment for Asthma.* Tarcher/Putnam, 2001.

————. *Headache Survival: The Holistic Medical Treatment for Migraine and Tension Headache.* Tarcher/Putnam, 2002.

Ivker, Robert; Anderson, Robert; Trivieri, Larry. *The Self-Care Guide to Holistic Medicine: Creating Optimal Health.* Tarcher/Putnam, 1999.

Joy, W. Brugh. *Joy's Way: A Map for the Transformational Journey.* Tarcher, 1979.

Keck, L. Robert. *Sacred Quest.* Chrysalis Books, 2000.

————. *Healing as a Sacred Path: A Story of Personal, Medical, and Spiritual Transformation.* Chrysalis Books, 2002.

Klein, Arthur; Sobel, Dava. *Backache Relief.* Timeless Books, 1985.

Kübler-Ross, Elisabeth. *On Death and Dying.* Scribner's, 1997.

Laskow, Leonard. *Healing with Love.* HarperSanFrancisco, 1992.

Luskin, Fred. *Forgive for Good.* HarperCollins, 2002.

Myss, Carolyn. *Anatomy of the Spirit.* Harmony Books, 1996.

Ornish, Dean. *Love & Survival.* HarperCollins, 1998.

Sarno, John. *Mind Over Back Pain.* Berkley Books, 1982.

Shannon, Scott. *Handbook of Complementary and Alternative Therapies in Mental Health.* Academic Press, 2001.

Siegel, Bernie. *Love, Medicine, and Miracles.* Harper & Row, 1986.

Sierpina, Victor. *Integrative Health Care.* F. A. Davis, 2001.

Trivieri, Larry. *The AHMA Guide to Holistic Health.* Wiley, 2001.

Vaillant, George. *Aging Well.* Little, Brown & Company, 2002.

Weil, Andrew. *Natural Health, Natural Medicine.* Houghton-Mifflin, 1990.

White, B. *Clinician's Guide to Spirituality and Chronic Illness.* McGraw-Hill, 2001.

White, Bowen. *Why Normal Isn't Healthy.* Hazelden, 2000.

INDEX

Index

Index

ABOUT THE AUTHOR

Robert S. Ivker, D.O.

Dr. Ivker is a holistic family physician, healer, teacher, and health consultant. He began practicing family medicine in Denver in 1972, after graduating from the Philadelphia College of Osteopathic Medicine. He completed a family practice residency at Mercy Medical Center in Denver and was certified by the American Board of Family Practice (ABFP) from 1975 to 1988. For the past sixteen years his holistic medical practice has focused on the treatment of chronic disease and the creation of optimal health. He is an Assistant Clinical Professor in the Department of Family Medicine and a Clinical Instructor in the Department of Otolaryngology at the University of Colorado School of Medicine. Dr. Ivker is a co-founder and president of the American Board of Holistic Medicine (ABHM) and co-creator of the first board certification examination in holistic medicine in December 2000. He was the president of the American Holistic Medical Association (AHMA) from 1996 to 1999. Along with the four editions of the best-selling *Sinus Survival: The Holistic Medical Treatment for Sinusitis, Allergies, and Colds,* Dr. Ivker is the co-author of *The Self-Care Guide to Holistic Medicine: Creating Optimal Health* and *Thriving: The Holistic Guide to Optimal Health for Men. Backache Survival* is part of a Survival Guide series that also includes *Arthritis Survival, Headache Survival,* and *Asthma Survival,* all published by Tarcher/Putnam in 2001 and 2002. He has been married for thirty-five years to Harriet, a psychiatric social worker; they have two daughters, Julie and Carin, and a son-in-law, Jeremy Dubin, and live in Littleton, Colorado.